Midwifery Practice:
Core Topics 1

First published 1996 by
MACMILLAN PRESS LTD
Houndmills, Basingstoke, Hampshire RG21 6XS
and London
Companies and representatives
throughout the world

ISBN 0–333–66320–9

A catalogue record for this book is available
from the British Library.

10   9   8   7   6   5   4   3   2   1
05   04   03   02   01   00   99   98   97   96

Typeset by Footnote Graphics, Warminster, Wilts
Printed and bound in Great Britain by
Mackays of Chatham PLC, Chatham, Kent

The editors, contributor and
publishers would like to thank
TY Khong *et al*, *The British Journal of
Obstetrics and Gynaecology*, and
Blackwell Science Publishers for permission
to use the illustrations on p. 135.

Dedicated to the memory of
ROSEMARY METHVEN
an outstanding midwife and researcher
who contributed to the success of the
first volume in this series,
and whose talents will be greatly missed
by her profession

Contents

Other volumes in the Midwifery Practice Series

■ **Volume 4   Midwifery practice: ISBN 0–333–57617–9 a research-based approach**

■ **Volume 5   Aspects of: ISBN 0–333–61956–0 midwifery practice**

Contributors to this volume

Tansy M. Cheston RGN, RM
Midwifery Sister, Silver Star Unit (High Risk Pregnancies), Oxford
At the Silver Star Unit, Tansy Cheston works closely with Professor
CWG Redman, a world authority on hypertension in pregnancy. The
unit is involved in many varied research projects connected with pre-
eclampsia and with attempting to find a cause for this distressing condition.

Rosemary Currell BA, MPhil, RN, RM
Research Associate, Centre for Health Informatics, University of Wales, Aberystwyth
A contributor to the first volume in the *Midwifery Practice* series, Rosemary
Currell has been working in health informatics for several years now,
and has special interests in maternity information, the development of
electronic patient records and confidentiality of health information.

Greta Curtis SRN, RM, ONC
*Specialist Nurse in Clinical Genetics, The Wessex Clinical Genetics Service,
Princess Anne Hospital, Southampton*
Greta Curtis is currently undertaking an MSc in Health Psychology at
Southampton University. Her research interests include improving com-
munication in clinical genetics, reproductive decision making and the
psychological effects of prenatal screening programmes.

Jane Denton RGN, RM
*Nursing Director, Multiple Births Foundation, Queen Charlotte's and Chelsea
Hospital, London*
Jane Denton had many years experience in a specialist infertility unit
before joining the Multiple Births Foundation where her work addresses
the many problems of multiple births arising from fertility treatment.
She is also a member of the Human Fertilisation and Embryology
Authority.

Kathleen King Licentiate (Belgium), MBA
Organisational Development Co-ordinator, Royal College of Nursing
Until August 1995, Kathleen King was lecturer in the management and

marketing of health services at the RCN Institute of Advanced Nursing Education. Her current role gives her the opportunity to apply theory to practice. She is also a visiting tutor at the London Business School.

Helen R Minns RM, RGN, BA(Hons), MTD
Lecturer–Practitioner In Midwifery, Oxford Brookes University/Oxford Team Midwives Women's Centre, The John Radcliffe Maternity Unit
Helen Minns has been involved in the education of midwives and family planning nurses for many years. She has a special interest in providing for the particular needs of young people and those with learning difficulties before, during and after childbirth.

Elsa Montgomery BSc(Hons), RGN, RM
Midwife, The Princess Anne Hospital, Southampton
Elsa Montgomery currently works part time as a midwife and has two small children. She contributed a chapter (on iron supplementation during pregnancy) to the fourth volume in the *Midwifery Practice* series.

Colin Rees Bsc(Hons), MSc, PGCE(FE)
Lecturer in Research, South East Wales Institute of Nursing and Midwifery Education, Caerleon, Gwent
Colin Rees has carried out research into a number of areas of midwifery, including antenatal education, and has written widely on midwifery topics. He teaches on several midwifery programmes, including the MSc in Reproduction and Health at the University of Wales College of Medicine, Cardiff.

Jennifer Wilson BSc (Hons), MSc, RGN, RM
Until recently, Research Midwife, Antenatal Care Project, UMDS, Guy's and St Thomas' Hospitals
Jenny Wilson's main research interest is in antenatal care; she has recently organised a large, randomised controlled trial comparing two schedules of antenatal visits. She has also worked with, and written about, the practices of traditional birth attendants. She is currently taking a short break from midwifery to have her first baby.

Foreword

The Winterton and Cumberlege Reports marked a new era for childbearing women and their families, and for the midwives who serve them. This new volume in the *Midwifery Practice* series, which will serve to relaunch the books, will be important to midwives as they move into the expanding territories of the new midwifery practice.

The series takes forward and deepens the arguements and theory underlying midwifery practice. Importantly, it draws on evidence and gives recommendations and a list for practice checks that will help to take theory into practice. Some of the chapters in this latest volume take the reader into topics that have not been explored before, but which are of fundamental importance if we are to serve the mixed needs of our population sensitively and effectively.

The chapters include in-depth examination of a variety of topics, covering clinical, educational and organisational aspects of care. The context of the book reflects the broad sphere of the practice of midwifery and concern for the physical, social and emotional aspects integral to midwifery practice.

Midwifery Practice: Core topics 1 will be a crucial resource for the modern midwife, student of midwifery and others, as we reform our maternity services.

Lesley Page
Queen Charlotte's Professor of Midwifery Practice
London

Preface

Core Topics 1, the sixth volume in the *Midwifery Practice* series, marks a watershed in our endeavours to provide practical, readable research-based texts for busy practitioners at an affordable price. We have listened to our 'consumers' and continue to strive to meet their varying needs in a rapidly changing care environment. Chapters retain the proven structure described below. The contributors address topical concerns as well as reviewing and updating some of the fundamental subject areas so important to midwifery. Again, we have sought a balance between core topics and contemporary issues in this volume, and we would welcome suggestions for future volumes.

Since beginning this series, it has become generally easier for midwives to access databases such as the Cochrane Collaborative Pregnancy and Childbirth Database and the MIRIAD Midwifery Research Database. However, practitioners do still benefit from having access to sound, well-referenced texts that address their needs and review a spread of relevant and up to date reference material. For some, this satisfies their needs, while for others it provides a springboard to the achievement of higher-level knowledge and research activity. As editors, we are committed to remaining firmly rooted in clinical practice, appealing both to those with limited time and to those wishing to investigate topics further.

Our contributors have delighted us with their meticulous work and willingness to meet our aspirations. Their critical appraisals of the literature will stimulate the reader seeking to evaluate different research approaches, and all midwives should find much to enhance their evidence-based practice. Women using the maternity services are increasingly knowledgeable and expect midwives to be properly equipped, both practically and academically. Getting the balance right is not easy, but we hope that this series will continue to make a useful contribution in this arena, encouraging education and practice to stay welded together and jointly driving clinical research.

Finally, we would like to thank our publishers, expecially our outstanding publishers' editor Richenda Milton-Thompson, and Carrie Walker who has recently joined us as copy editor.

JA, VL, SR

■ Common structure of the chapters

In fulfilment of the aims of the series, each chapter follows a common structure:

1. The introduction offers a digest of the contents;

2. 'It is assumed that you are already aware of the following ...' establishes the prerequisite knowledge and experience assumed of the reader;

3. The main body of the chapter then reviews and analyses the most appropriate and important research literature currently available;

4. The 'Recommendations for clinical practice' offer suggestions for sound clinical practice, based on the author's interpretation of the literature;

5. The 'Practice check' enables professionals to examine their own practice and the principles and policies influencing their work;

6. Bibliographic sources are covered under 'References' and 'Suggested further reading'.

■ Suggested further reading on research

Burnard P, Morrison P 1994 Nursing research in action: developing basic skills, 2nd edn. Macmillan, Basingstoke

Cormack DFS (ed.) 1996 The research process in nursing, 3rd edn. Blackwell Science, Oxford

Couchman W, Dawson J 1995 Nursing and healthcare research, 2nd edn. Scutari Press, London

Distance Learning Centre packages 1988–94 Research awareness: a programme for nurses, midwives and health visitors, Units 1–11. South Bank University, London

Hicks C 1990 Research and statistics: a practical introduction for nurses. Prentice Hall, Hemel Hempstead

Polit DF, Hungler BP 1995 Nursing research: principles and methods, 5th edn. JB Lippincott, Philadelphia

Chapter 1

The organisation of maternity care

Rosemary Currell

The past 10 years have seen a proliferation of different patterns of maternity care, all aiming to provide women and their babies with safe, efficient care that is emotionally pleasing to them and that meets their social and domestic needs. All those responsible for bringing about a change in the maternity services do so in the belief that this particular change will bring some measure of benefit to women and their families. It should be recognised, however, that the circumstances that have brought each pattern of care into being, and the driving forces that take it forward and bring about its evolution, are all very different and very complex. The driving forces for change in the maternity services include social change, national politics, professional interests, advances in health care and the personal experiences of families and health care professionals. Academic research has its place but may more usually be found as a tool used within one of these arenas rather than as a pressure in its own right. We therefore need to look very carefully at the evidence used to support any particular development or change in the provision of maternity care. We need to consider not only the validity and reliability of the research itself, but also how it is being used, whose arguments and theories it is being used to support, and for what ends.

Opposing views about how maternity care should be organised can be held equally sincerely by different groups and individuals, all believing that their way will be 'best' for mothers and babies, and there are indeed many ways of fulfilling the same ends. However, it should also be remembered that different situations require different solutions, and the challenge in the organisation of maternity care is to decide the most appropriate means for the service in every area. Clearly what is right for a deprived inner city area with a mobile population is unlikely to be exactly right for a very scattered, but stable, rural population. The care required by a healthy 27-year-old having her second baby will not be the same as that needed by a 38-year-old who has had a renal transplant and is now expecting her first child.

In this chapter, the issues affecting the organisation of maternity care, the research evidence for different methods of providing care, and the questions those responsible for any part of the service should ask, will all be explored.

■ It is assumed that you are already aware of the following:

- The history of the maternity services in the UK;
- The way in which maternity services are organised in your area, and the rationale for any recent changes or developments;
- The House of Commons Health Committee Report on the Maternity Services (1992) and the *Changing childbirth* report (DoH 1993).

■ How should the organisation of maternity care be assessed?

While the provision of maternity services is a matter of universal concern, the current WHO Safe Motherhood initiative (Kwast 1991), which aims to reduce maternal mortality in the Third World by 50 per cent within a decade, stands in stark contrast to some of the preoccupations of Western policy makers. Every maternity care service must be seen in its own social and economic setting but must also be examined in the same way as any other type of health service provision, and therefore be evaluated for its clinical effectiveness, its efficiency, its cost effectiveness, its accessibility, its acceptability and its equity.

The fact that this book includes a chapter on the organisation of maternity care is an indication that the organisation of care is neither a straightforward matter nor a constant within the maternity services. In earlier times, with only the village midwife and the local doctor available to provide care, the issues of how and when to intervene, the efficacy of various treatments, professional demarcation lines, access to services and ability to pay were all open to debate, as they are now. However, because care was only offered by these two professionals, and took place predominantly in women's own homes, the actual organisation of care was very simple. There were very few institutions to manage and very few care providers with whom to communicate. In today's highly complex and ever-changing health services, the ability to communicate, and to have accurate information available at all the points where care is provided, is essential to the provision of effective, efficient and acceptable health care.

■ Changing childbirth

Maternity care cannot be separated from its political context and has always been subject to direction and control by representatives of the Church or state (see for example Donnison 1977), and the 20th century has been no exception (Currell 1990). The midwifery profession is itself the subject of an act of parliament in the UK, and the fight for the legalisation of midwifery in North America is certainly centred around power and politics.

It is accepted in democratic states that government should be concerned with the health and welfare of its citizens, and that public funds and resources should be used responsibly for the good of all. In the UK, the political ideologies underlying the reforms of the NHS have had an effect on the provision of maternity services. Providers of services in areas in which women have real choice about where to have their babies have been forced to take the wishes of their consumers seriously and attempt to provide what they think their customers want. The purchaser–provider split has encouraged health authorities to look at the value of the services they are purchasing for their populations. Ensuring that services are acceptable to consumers, effective and efficient must be to the good of all concerned. None of this should present any difficulties for the maternity services, but politics is essentially about power, about who can be the most persuasive and about good intentions, rather than about rational argument.

The provision of maternity services has been the subject of a number of government reports during the second half of the 20th century (Currell 1990). Each of these has had a significant impact on the service, and it has been the most recent UK government reports on the maternity services that have quite overtly been the driving force for much of the current change. Select Committees of the House of Commons have been convened to consider various aspects of the maternity services. These committees invite 'experts' to advise them, others with an interest from various backgrounds are invited to submit evidence, the committee members visit suggested maternity units and anyone else who chooses is free to submit evidence. Professor Philip Steer, in a commentary on the House of Commons Health Committee Report (Steer 1992), suggests that committees will ask for scientific evidence related to the subject in question but that the evidence from which the final report is drawn is largely opinion (albeit well informed) and the strongly held beliefs of those who take the trouble to write to the committee. It may be difficult for the reader to distinguish between recommendations based on hard evidence and those based on opinion, with no foundation in fact. This can have serious consequences. For example, the House of Commons Social Services Committee Report on Perinatal and Maternal Mortality (1980) (the Short Report) recommended that 'An increasing number of mothers should be delivered in large units ... home delivery should be phased out further.' The work of Campbell and Macfarlane (1994) shows that there is no clear causal relationship between the increase in the number of hospital births and the concurrent decrease in perinatal mortality, yet many small maternity units (often providing the 'humanised' care the committee also recommends) have been closed, and many individual pregnant women and consultant obstetricians have argued painfully about the advisability or otherwise of a home birth. The same committee also recommended that 'Continuous recording of the fetal heart rate should increasingly become part of the surveillance of all babies during labour.' However, rigorous trials brought together by the National Perinatal Epidemiology Unit (Chalmers *et al* 1989) have shown no scientific basis for this practice. The Committee did, of course, make many other important recommendations, which have benefitted the maternity services in the intervening years, but this should serve as a warning to any who might be tempted to take all the findings and recommendations of government reports as incontrovertible.

The House of Commons Health Committee Report (1992) met with perhaps a more vigorous and mixed reaction than preceding reports on the maternity services, and its impact on maternity services in the UK has been dramatic. The report may come to be seen as the culmination of the natural childbirth versus high-technology childbirth, and the consumer versus medical professions, battles that have raged throughout the Western world over the past 30 years. In broad terms, the report appears to sanction a shift in the balance of power, from the traditionally powerful and predominantly male medical profession to the previously submissive, female consumers and their advocates, the midwives. To have government take the views of women and families seriously in this way, and to perceive the need to shift from perinatal and neonatal mortality and morbidity as the only outcomes of significance in the maternity services, has to be welcomed. As with all revolutionary documents, however, there is the risk that the case may have been overstated, that the protagonists, in order to win their point, have made claims that cannot be fully substantiated, and that those who now feel that their position has been vindicated may throw caution to the wind in their zeal to accomplish long-cherished dreams, despite the fact that the Committee stated, 'We do not wish this report to mark another extreme in the swing of the pendulum' (House of Commons Health Committee 1992: 1xxx).

The House of Commons Health Committee comments on a wide range of clinical and policy issues in maternity care, and on the need for reliable research. It makes recommendations about the link between social deprivation and poor outcomes for mothers and babies, as the Short Committee (House of Commons Social Services Committee 1980) had done before it, and points to a lack of research evidence on the adequacy of benefit levels, which are of course truly political concerns. The House of Commons Health Committee properly highlights the lack of research evidence – on postnatal care, on interventions in intrapartum care and on the cost of various organisational patterns of care provision – and the way in which research evidence has, in practice, been ignored in the provision of antenatal care. However, in the development of its major themes, the Committee shows unhelpful inconsistencies. For example, it pursues the ideology of continuity of care throughout the document, with only one reference to the research evidence supporting continuity of care. It quotes from *Effective care in pregnancy and childbirth* (Chalmers *et al* 1989), in which it is stated that any form of care that fails to provide continuity in pregnancy and childbirth should be abandoned. In her 1993 review of 'Continuity of caregivers during pregnancy and childbirth' for the Pregnancy & Childbirth Module of the Cochrane Database of Systematic Reviews, Hodnett found only one acceptable trial and concluded that further research on continuity of care needs to be undertaken before undertaking major restructuring of the service in an attempt to provide continuity. It is, perhaps, unfortunate that this information was not available to the House of Commons Health Committee in 1992.

Another major theme throughout the report is that of control: control for women, and also control amongst the professions. The Committee makes a number of references to disagreements between the professions, which may be entirely justified. However, in the confusion of its recommendations, the Committee has hardly eased the path of agreement between the supposed protagonists. The Committee acknowledges the contribution that GPs make to continuity of care for women and the need for women to have choice of by whom and where their antenatal care is provided, yet it recommends 'a radical reappraisal of the current system of shared care with a presumption in favour of its abandonment'. This is, to say the least, unhelpful in its inconsistency. The Committee's recommendations for the development of midwifery care in initiatives such as midwifery-led units are to be welcomed, but all this has to be seen in conjunction with another of the Committee's major themes – choice for women themselves – which could be limited rather than enhanced by some of these proposals.

It was left to the professions themselves to redress the balance in their responses to the report. In its response, the Royal College of Obstetricians and Gynaecologists (RCOG) (1992) stressed the need for women to have access to the care of midwives, obstetricians and GPs, and midwives also stressed the determination of the professions to work together (Brain 1992). The Royal Colleges of Obstetricians and Gynaecologists, General Practitioners and Midwives produced a joint document in which they welcomed the findings of the Committee but stressed the importance of collaboration, stating that each profession has a well-defined role in maternity care. In this joint statement, they also took the view that as midwives are the major providers of practical maternity care, and if women are to have continuity of care, midwifery services will need to be reorganised to provide this, and suggested that this could be achieved by midwives having identified caseloads.

The government's response to the House of Commons Health Committee Report was to set up the Expert Maternity Group under the chairmanship of Lady Cumberlege. *Changing childbirth* (DoH 1993) is the result of this group's deliberations; it begins with a statement of the 'Principles of good maternity care', of which the first is that 'The woman must be the focus of maternity care.' The House of Commons Health Committee (1992) spoke of the need to 'humanise' the maternity services, as its predecessors had also done. It is hard to believe that midwives and the other professions involved in the maternity services need to have these principles spelt out and that 'care' in the maternity services still cannot be taken for granted.

One of the difficulties of this report (DoH 1993) is its uneasy mix of attempting to promote individualised care, while at the same time proposing organisational change that could appear prescriptive. What is required is to attempt to provide each woman with what she needs and what she wants, and to recognise that this is going to be infinitely variable and that needs and wants are not always compatible. This is what woman-centred care really means. Just as we are told that women *want* continuity of care, there are women who tell us that they *want* to have more of their antenatal care at the hospital, and women who tell us that they would *like* to see the consultant obstetrician on every visit. None of these requests can be supported by sound research evidence for their benefits, but to deny the possibility of any of these options would be to restrict women's choice. It is just as important for those professionals who advocate a 'natural' and open approach to childbirth, as it is for those who take a more technological approach, to listen to what each woman wants for herself and her baby. It is more important than ever for professional practice and advice to women to be founded wherever possible on sound evidence, even though women and their partners must be free to make their own choices. Choice and freedom for women requires professionals at all points on the technology/natural childbirth continuum to be clear about the benefits and consequences of one mode of care rather than another.

The Expert Maternity Group (DoH 1993) has explicitly advocated the development of the midwifery profession and the full use of midwifery skills by all midwives. The misuse and waste of midwifery skills and expertise was demonstrated by Robinson *et al* (1983) in their research on the role and responsibilities of the midwife more than a decade ago, so this official commitment to midwifery is long overdue. However, in their enthusiasm for midwifery and with their underlying adherence to the concept of continuity of midwifery care, this Group has also produced some very muddled thinking on the roles of the various members of the maternity care team and the possible organisational arrangements. This is particularly unfortunate because it elicited a far less measured response from the RCOG (1993) than the House of Commons Report (1992) had done. The RCOG agreed with the need for change but was unhappy that major change was being suggested without an objective review of the evidence. Once any group feels it has to take up a defensive position, working co-operatively for change immediately becomes more difficult. If women are to experience more sensitive care through reform of the organisation of the service, midwives, GPs and obstetricians will now need to be very sensitive to the needs of their colleagues as well as to those of their clients.

■ Patterns of maternity care

□ Clinical outcomes

If we believe that the way in which maternity care is provided makes a significant difference to outcomes for mothers and babies – and the recent UK government reports and subsequent activity suggest that we do – we must subject the organisation of maternity care to the same kind of rigorous evaluation that is applied to other aspects of clinical activity. The work of the National Perinatal Epidemiology Unit and the publication of *Effective care in pregnancy and childbirth* (Chalmers *et al* 1989) have shown that there can be no complacency or uninformed use of treatments and interventions in maternity care, and the organisation of that care should be no exception. In arguing the case for randomised controlled trials in perinatal medicine, Lilford (1989) warns that very few treatments are without monetary or human cost, and suggests that trials should be used not only to control the introduction of new practices, but also to prevent established and useful methods from being abandoned.

The Expert Maternity Group (DoH 1993) describes safety as the foundation of good maternity care, and the basic measures of perinatal mortality and morbidity are therefore seen as important components of the evaluation of the organisation of care. A study by Mascarenhas *et al* (1992), comparing perinatal outcome in England and Wales with that in France, shows similar perinatal outcomes in similar populations, with very different systems of care providers, different levels of provision of antenatal care and different applications of obstetric technology. This is helpful in a review of different patterns of maternity care as it raises two issues: first, very different patterns of care can produce very similar results, and second, as stated by Lilford (1989), where the standard of a particular outcome is already very high, it is going to be difficult to demonstrate a further significant improvement whatever the intervention (or change in the pattern of care).

The outcomes chosen as measures of the effectiveness of different kinds of organisation should be wider than those for measuring more specific interventions and may include measures of social and emotional outcome. Most of the patterns of care that have emerged recently have centred around midwifery care, and there is the suggestion that mid-wifery care is likely to be not only more 'human', but also less technical than obstetric care. For example, the studies by Klein *et al* (1983, 1985) showed a difference in the use of technology by hospital-based and com-munity-based midwives caring for low-risk women. While a reduction in the use of technology may not be the explicit reason for the promotion of midwifery-based care, that expectation may exist, making it difficult to determine exactly what is being evaluated in some studies – intervention and the use of technology, or the pattern of care.

The studies describing changes in the patterns of delivery of mid-wifery care are largely concerned with demonstrating that it is possible for midwives to undertake the full care of women with low-risk pregnancies and achieve outcomes of perinatal and maternal mortality and morbidity as good as those achieved with conventional obstetric care. The schemes vary considerably in the patterns of care they provide and in their research design, making it difficult to compare them and draw conclusions about their outcomes. Where clinical outcomes for the schemes have been measured, most studies have looked at factors such as interventions in labour, length of labour, use of analgesia, Apgar scores and admission of babies to special care baby units. In the debate stimulated by the report of the Aberdeen Midwife Managed Delivery Unit (Hundley *et al* 1994), it was pointed out that the sample size required to show a differ-ence in serious perinatal morbidity for different kinds of care was very much larger than that in this study, and that a single trial of sufficient size might not be feasible (Brocklehurst *et al* 1995). The same is, of course, true for the even rarer events of maternal and perinatal mortality, so that proving statistically that midwifery care is as safe as or safer than obstetric care is beyond the scope of the studies found in the literature to date.

☐ **Client satisfaction**

The need to widen the concept of clinical outcomes has been noted, together with the consumers' concerns about the acceptability and 'humanness' of maternity care. The current debate about choice for women, and the introduction of formal competition into the NHS, means that service providers are now forced to try to provide consumers with the kind of service they want (as most health care professionals have, with varying degrees of success, always attempted to do), and to consider seriously the acceptability, accessibility and equity of their services. The Department of Health (DoH) has considered the issue sufficiently important to produce the document *Assessing women's views of maternity services* (Mason 1990). Client satisfaction is a term much used and abused in the health service today, and it has been shown to be a multifaceted concept. To ensure that it is embedded in the equally complex organisational structures of modern maternity care is no simple matter.

The maternity care schemes introduced in recent years have all explicitly aimed to improve women's satisfaction with care in one way or another, predominantly by improving continuity of midwifery care (see for example Flint *et al* 1989; Frohlich & Edwards 1989; Lester & Farrow 1989; Watson 1990). The evaluation of some maternity care schemes has included the assessment of women's satisfaction with the care they received, but the rigour of the research methodology of these studies varies considerably, ranging from a full statistical analysis of the St George's randomised controlled trial (Flint *et al* 1989) to the Bristol study (Ward & Frohlich 1994), which had no control group for the mothers' opinions. It is surprising just how few outcome and evaluation reports of these schemes have been published, considering the enthusiasm for reorganising maternity care in the past few years (Wraight *et al* 1993). Wraight *et al* found that only one third of established team midwifery schemes had sought to assess women's views of their care, and only one third of discontinued schemes had been formally evaluated. It must be significant also that, in commissioning the 'Mapping Team Midwifery' study, the DoH did not include an analysis of outcome measures of evaluations of the schemes in its objectives, even though the purpose of the study was to help those responsible for the provision of services in their development work. It is not possible to know whether the lack of reported evaluations is due to the reluctance of midwives to publish their work, to dissatisfaction with the findings or to whether schemes have not been formally evaluated at all.

Judith Lumley, in her paper 'Assessing satisfaction with childbirth' (1985), suggests that soft outcomes are often ignored because they are difficult and, she says, 'confront us with hard problems, problems of person, place, population and time. In other words, who is assessing satisfaction? *Whose* satisfaction is in question? *Where* is the assessment taking place? *When* is it being carried out? *How* is satisfaction being assessed?' (Lumley 1985: 141–5). These are very pertinent questions for service providers, health professionals, lay representatives, service purchasers and researchers, who all want accurate knowledge of what makes a maternity service satisfying for its consumers. They are questions that should be asked of any study aiming to describe women's satisfaction with their care. For example, was it the midwives giving care to the women who gave out the questionnaires about the team midwifery scheme, and if so are the responses coloured by the desire of the women to please the midwives? The aims of many new patterns of maternity care are to improve the use of skills and provide job satisfaction for midwives. Who derives most emotional satisfaction from a particular pattern of care – mother or midwife? Is a woman's account of her care in labour and delivery the same if her husband is present at the interview and was present at the birth as it would be if she talked about it on her own? Does the assessment take place in the busy hospital ward or clinic or at the woman's own kitchen table, and what differences might be expected between these settings? Lumley suggests that assessment too close to the experience of childbirth will not be accurate, and that some time after the first 6 months will produce a more honest response from mothers. The methods used to assess satisfaction can be very crude or very complex, and Lumley says (1985: 143), 'It is as if the forced choice method cannot do justice to the range and complexity of the human feelings involved.'

Another serious problem in any client satisfaction survey is the characteristics of those who do not respond to questionnaires or who cannot be traced for interviews. In her study of women's perceptions of their care, Cartwright (1987) shows that women who were young, single, non-Caucasian and not living in owner-occupied homes were less likely than other mothers to describe the care they received during labour and delivery as 'very kind and understanding'. These are the women who are most disadvantaged in society, most mobile, most likely to have difficulties with language and communication, and therefore most likely not to be included in the final outcome of studies unless extra effort has been made to contact them. Those most likely to encounter difficulties with the maternity services, and probably the most in need, may therefore be the group least likely to make their views known.

The recent reports and discussion about the maternity services have shown that there are generally held and accepted beliefs about what women want in their maternity care. These are centered around the House of Commons Health Committee's (1992) principles of continuity, choice and control, and the 'Indicators for success' in *Changing childbirth* (DoH 1993) also focus providers very specifically on a limited range of factors within the whole gamut and complexity of the maternity services. This creates a situation in which it is possible for investigators inadvertently to continue to reinforce the current, largely unsubstantiated, view of what women want. It is quite reasonable to ask women about specific topics, but they also need to be allowed to express views about issues that they might consider to be *more* important.

Some writers (for example Seguin *et al* 1989; Green *et al* 1990; Brown & Lumley 1994) draw attention to the fact that the distinction needs to be made between women's satisfaction with their birth experience and their satisfaction with the care they have received. Determining satisfaction with maternity care is thus shown to be a highly complicated issue, in which the underlying concepts need to be much better understood.

☐ **Choice**

Clearly no single pattern of care is going to be right for every woman, and if a service is to be acceptable and accessible, it must also offer choice, as the House of Commons Health Committee (1992) and Expert Maternity Group (DoH 1993) so strongly assert. However, the introduction of new schemes has in some cases meant that previously successful schemes have had to cease, thus restricting women's choice. The fact that so many of the new patterns for maternity care appear to depend on the concept of risk creates the danger of excluding some women from a pattern of care, in just the same way that multiparous women at low risk in the 1950s were expected to have a home delivery (Campbell & Macfarlane 1994). Equity in the provision of service is thus compromised. There is a danger, too, that the fact that the Expert Maternity Group's indicators are not evidence-based will soon be forgotten as they become part of the received wisdom of the maternity services, and they could become as difficult to change as the traditional pattern of antenatal visits (Hall *et al* 1980; RCOG 1982), which was laid down in a very similar way.

☐ **Effective use of resources**

While choice for women in the overall pattern of care they receive should always be a consideration, finite resources and local conditions are always going to mean that choice must be circumscribed. All the health services in the Western world are grappling with the problems of how to make the best use of finite resources in the face of infinite demand for health care, and the maternity services cannot expect special pleading. In the UK, the most recent NHS reforms, with the 'purchaser–provider split', are one response to this problem and have meant that the maternity services are subject to far greater examination than ever before. Competitiveness between maternity units has always existed in an informal way, but has now become a serious issue in some areas of the country, particularly in large conurbations. Very little work has been done to date on the comparative costs of different patterns of maternity care, although some studies are now underway (for example Page *et al* 1994). Wraight *et al* (1993) found almost no information on the relative costs of team midwifery, and the NHS Management Executive study team (1993) also found very little reliable evidence on the comparative costs of different patterns of care. Some studies of the provision of antenatal care have specifically looked at the use of resources and at their costs (for example Twaddle & Harper 1992; Tucker *et al* 1994).

■ Maternity services and the health care professionals

Successful interdisciplinary working is a major factor in the provision of clinically effective maternity care, as the majority of women in the Western world receive at least part of their care from members of the medical profession. What is very much still open to debate is how the balance of care between midwives and doctors should be achieved. The debate should be informed by the needs of women for the care and skills of each professional at any particular point in pregnancy, labour or delivery, or postpartum, by the evidence of how that need can best be met, by the judgement of each profession on how they can most effectively provide that care, and by the need to provide a flexible service giving women choice wherever possible.

Two other issues appear to be in danger of being lost in this debate. First, women at high risk in pregnancy, and those with special needs requiring medical help, need every bit as much midwifery care as do their sisters considered as being at low risk (see Chapter 3 in this volume). Patterns of maternity care that provide a different quality of service for different groups of women cannot be defended. The second issue is that midwives do not have the monopoly on continuity of care: doctors, too, like to build up trusting and satisfying relationships with their patients. Why should it be any easier for a doctor than it is for a midwife to meet a woman for the first time in a crisis? Doctors, just as much as midwives, need to see the outcomes for their patients in order to learn and progress.

The way in which maternity care is organised must have a major impact not only on those who receive the service, but also on those who provide it. Questions of acceptability should be asked from their point of view, as well as that of their clients, as a service that cannot attract or retain staff will never be efficient or fully effective.

However care is organised, it is clear that women need kind, sensitive, intelligent and purposeful care from every midwife and every health professional they meet, whatever the setting and whether they meet once only or become good friends.

■ Recommendations for clinical practice in the light of currently available evidence

1. Research is needed into the concept of continuity of care and exactly what care it is that women want when they ask for continuity.

2. Any reorganisation of maternity care should be carefully evaluated before and after implementation. Particular care should be taken that popular existing schemes are not abandoned without being adequately replaced.

3. Any proposed reorganisation of care should not benefit one group of its clients more than another.

4. The views of women from all sections of society and with special needs should be sought when considering major change in a local maternity service.

5. Any proposed reorganisation should take into account the professional and personal needs of all members of the maternity care team.

■ Practice check

- Do you know how your clients travel to the various places where their antenatal care is provided, and how easy or difficult those journeys are?

- Do you know what it is that women particularly appreciate about the care they receive in your unit, and what they find difficult or unsatisfactory?

- Do you know whether your clients have all the information they need for making decisions about their maternity care, and where they find it?

- Do you discuss maternity care with your medical and other paramedical colleagues and try to understand it from their perspective?

■ References

Brain M 1992 The Maternity Services Report. Midwives Chronicle   105(1257): 314–16

Brocklehurst P, Macfarlane A, Dudley L, Garcia J, Elbourne D 1995 Conclusions are not supported by results. British Medical Journal   310: 805–7 (letter)

Brown S, Lumley J 1994 Satisfaction with care in labor and birth: a survey of 790 Australian women. Birth   21: 4–13

Campbell R, Macfarlane A 1994 Where to be born? The debate and the evidence, 2nd edn. National Perinatal Epidemiology Unit, Radcliffe Infirmary, Oxford

Cartwright A 1987 Who are maternity services kind to? What is kindness? Midwife, Health Visitor and Community Nurse   23(1): 21–4

Chalmers I, Enkin M, Keirse M (eds) 1989 Effective care in pregnancy and childbirth. Oxford University Press, Oxford

Currell R 1990 The organisation of maternity care. In: Alexander J, Levy V, Roch S (eds) Antenatal care: a research-based approach. Macmillan, Basingstoke, Ch 2, p20–41

Department of Health 1993 Changing childbirth. Report of the Expert Maternity Group. HMSO, London

Donnison J 1977 Midwives and medical men: a history of inter-professional rivalries and women's rights. Heinemann, London

Flint C, Poulgeneris P, Grant A 1989 The 'Know Your Midwife' scheme – a randomised trial of continuity of care by a team of midwives. Midwifery 5: 11–16

Frohlich J, Edwards S 1989 Team midwifery for everyone – building on the 'Know Your Midwife' scheme. Midwives Chronicle   102(1214): 66–70

Green J, Coupland V, Kitzinger J 1990 Expectations, experiences and psychological outcomes of childbirth: a prospective study of 825 women. Birth   17: 15–23

Hall M, Chng P, MacGillivray I 1980 Is routine antenatal care worthwhile? Lancet i: 78–80

Hodnett E 1993 Continuity of caregivers during pregnancy and childbirth. In Enkin M, Keirse M, Renfrew M, Neilson J (eds) Pregnancy and Childbirth Module, Cochrane Database of Systematic Reviews. Update Software, Oxford

House of Commons Social Services Committee 1980 Report on Perinatal and Neonatal Mortality (the Short Report). HMSO, London

House of Commons Health Committee 1992 Second Report, Maternity Services (the Winterton Committee Report). HMSO, London

Hundley V, Cruickshank FM, Lang GD, Glazener CMA, Milne JM, Turner M, Blyth D, Mollison J, Donaldson C 1994 Midwife managed delivery unit: a randomised controlled comparison with consultant led care. British Medical Journal   309: 1400–4

Klein M, Lloyd I, Redman C, Bull M, Turnbull A 1983 A comparison of low-risk women booked for delivery in two different systems of care – shared care and GPU. British Journal of Obstetrics and Gynaecology   90 (2): 118–28

Klein M, Elbourne D, Lloyd I 1985 A prospective study comparing the experience of low risk women booked for delivery in two systems of maternity care. Royal College of General Practitioners, London

Kwast B 1991 Safe motherhood: a challenge to midwifery practice. World Health Forum   12: 1–24

Lester C, Farrow S 1989 An evaluation of the Rhondda 'Know Your Midwives' scheme. The first year's deliveries. Institute of Health Care Evaluation, University of Wales College of Medicine, Cardiff

Lilford R 1989 Evaluating new treatments and diagnostic technologies in obstetrics. International Journal of Technology Assessment in Health Care 5: 459–72

Lumley J 1985 Assessing satisfaction with childbirth. Birth   12(3): 141–5

Mascarenhas L, Eliot B W, MacKenzie IZ 1992 A comparison of perinatal outcome, antenatal and intrapartum care between England and Wales, and France. British Journal of Obstetrics and Gynaecology   99:955–8

Mason V 1990 Assessing women's views of maternity services. HMSO, London

NHS Management Executive 1993 A study of midwife and GP led maternity units. HMSO, London

Page L, Wilkins R, Bridges A, Garcia J, Hewison J, Lathlean J, Lilford R, Newburn M, Piercey J, Stevens T 1994 Evaluating innovations in the organisation of midwifery practice. In Page L (ed.) Effective group practice in midwifery. Blackwell Scientific, Oxford, p174–88

President of the Royal College of Obstetricians and Gynaecologists, President of the Royal College of Midwives, Chairman of the Council of the Royal College of General Practitioners 1992 Maternity care in the new NHS: a joint approach. RCOG, RCM, RCGP, London

Robinson S, Golden J, Bradley S 1983 A study of the role and responsibilities of the midwife. NERU Report No. 1, Nursing Research Unit, King's College, University of London

Royal College of Obstetricians and Gynaecologists 1982 Report of the RCOG Working Party on antenatal and intrapartum care. RCOG, London

Royal College of Obstetricians and Gynaecologists 1993 Press Release, 6.8.1993, Changing childbirth, Report of the Expert Group on the Maternity Services, RCOG, London

Seguin L, Therrien R, Champagne F, Larouche D 1989 The components of women's satisfaction with maternity care. Birth 16: 109–13

Steer P 1992 The House of Commons Committee Report on the Maternity Services. A personal view. British Journal of Obstetrics and Gynaecology 99: 445–6

Tucker J, Florey C, Howie P, McIllwaine G, Hall M 1994 Is antenatal care apportioned according to obstetric risk? The Scottish antenatal care study. Journal of Public Health Medicine 16(1): 60–70

Twaddle S, Harper V 1992 An economic evaluation of daycare in the management of hypertension in pregnancy. British Journal of Obstetrics and Gynaecology 99: 459–63

Ward P, Frohlich J 1994 Team midwifery in Bristol. MIDIRS Digest 4(2): 149–51

Watson P 1990 Report on the Kidlington Team Midwifery Scheme. National Institute for Nursing, Radcliffe Infirmary, Oxford

Wraight A, Ball J, Seccombe I, Stock J 1993 Mapping team midwifery. Institute of Manpower Studies, Brighton

Chapter 2

Preconception care

Greta Curtis

The philosophy of preconception care is to increase the public's awareness of the importance of improving the health of both partners prior to a pregnancy. Preconception care is their mental and physical preparation for childbearing and is advocated as an approach to improve pregnancy outcomes (Jack & Culpepper 1990).

Although the concept of preconception care may be new to some midwives, the elements are very familiar to many others and can be effectively delivered by them. Midwives are providers of high-quality, individualised care who place an emphasis on appropriate risk assessment, health promotion and psychological support. They have, to a large extent, always provided preconception care outside the domain of a preconception clinic.

Most women are aware of the cause and effect relationship between 'risky' lifestyle behaviours (that is, smoking, drugs and alcohol) and perinatal outcome. However, the majority of women who become pregnant do not seek prenatal care and advice until the middle of the first trimester. By that time, organogenesis is well advanced and it may have already been affected by the client's lifestyle, including not only the healthy, but also the unhealthy, behaviours. Knowledge of preconception care has the potential of changing behaviour, modifying risks and improving the health status of potential parents. The target clientele for preconception advice should be all individuals of reproductive age, particularly women who are contemplating a pregnancy in the near future and teenage schoolchildren.

A peril of preconception care is that it assumes a planned pregnancy. However, in a study by Adams *et al* (1993), it was estimated that only 60 per cent of all pregnancies were planned. The study group self-reported their involvement in 'risky behaviours', that is, smoking, alcohol and drug taking, at the time of conception. Mothers of unintended pregnancies were more likely to have an indication for preconception care, in that they participated more often in one or more of these 'behaviours', than were mothers with planned pregnancies. There might possibly be a decline in the number of unplanned pregnancies if the use of family planning services were increased and information about preconception health practices were included in health education programmes. This would need to be fully evaluated prospectively to examine the uptake of preconception care and its effect on clients' health status and the outcome of the pregnancies.

The aspects of preconception care that will be included in this chapter are:

- Nutrition and diet;
- Pre-existing medical conditions: epilepsy, diabetes and phenylketonuria;
- Risky behaviours: smoking and alcohol (social and illicit drug use is not included);
- Family planning;
- Screening for health;
- Genetic counselling.

■ It is assumed that you are already aware of the following:

- The physiology of the menstrual cycle, including hormonal control, phases and possible variations, in order to assist women with awareness of their own fertility;
- The processes of meiosis, fertilisation and mitotic cell division;
- The process of spermatogenesis, the transport of semen to the seminal vesicles and the content of the normal sample of ejaculate;
- The formation of the blastocyst;
- Embryonic and fetal development, including the adverse factors that may interfere with normal cell differentiation;
- The aetiology of diabetes, epilepsy and phenylketonuria.

■ Diet and nutrition

An overview of the principles of good nutrition during pregnancy and lactation has been given elsewhere (Spedding *et al* 1995). It is, however, ideal for a woman's nutritional status to be good *before* conception takes place.

A woman's nutritional status may have profound repercussions upon a reproductive outcome, affecting the woman's fertility, the chance of early spontaneous abortion and the occurrence of neural tube defects. The use of the body mass index (BMI) to assess nutritional status prior to pregnancy should ascertain overweight or underweight women. The body mass index is calculated as weight (kg) divided by height in metres squared (m^2). Those with eating disorders, for example bulimia and anorexia nervosa, should also be identified. Once problems are identified, nutritional counselling and in some cases treatment of an underlying emotional condition can be initiated (Jack & Culpepper 1991).

The onset of menarche is delayed if fat stores are low, and if they are diminished after the onset of menarche, the menses are likely to become irregular and infrequent and possibly stop (Frisch & McArthur 1974). Dancers, athletes and women with anorexia nervosa show evidence of markedly diminished fertility (Warren 1980). Self-imposed weight loss by dieting has been shown to be a common cause of infertility and amenorrhoea in more than 50 per cent of women attending some infertility clinics (Haller 1992).

Food shortages and famines during World War II demonstrated the disastrous effect that a poor maternal nutritional state has on a fetus. During the 'Dutch hunger winter' of 1944–5, the highest incidence of neonatal deaths, caused by congenital abnormalities, was apparent if the woman conceived around the time of the food shortage (Wynn & Wynn 1981). The 'Dutch hunger winter' caused a fall in the live birth rate of about 50 per cent, partly due to an increase in the number of stillbirths and early miscarriages.

Underweight women who gain little weight in pregnancy are particularly at risk of having both preterm and low birthweight babies (Abrams & Laros 1986; Abrams & Neuman 1989). Attitudes and feelings regarding weight gain during pregnancy, its impact on the health of the baby, and the mother's perception of how the weight gain influences her own body image were investigated in a study by Copper *et al* (1995). The study demonstrated that prepregnant obese women tended to have negative attitudes towards weight gain in pregnancy, the lowest weight gain but the heaviest babies. Thin women had higher attitude scores and a higher mean weight gain in pregnancy but the lightest babies. Preconception nutritional advice and interventions, leading to an increased prepregnancy weight gain and a more desirable BMI in thin women, may play an important part in reducing the incidence of low birthweight babies (Copper *et al* 1995) and ultimately perinatal morbidity and mortality. Studies are needed to evaluate this.

☐ **Iron and vitamin supplementation**

A detailed discussion of the recent research literature relating to iron and vitamin supplementation is beyond the scope of this chapter, and the reader is referred to Montgomery (1993).

☐ **Folic acid supplementation**

It has been recognised for some time that the use of vitamin supplementation has had a protective effect against the incidence of neural tube defects (NTDs) among women who have already experienced an NTD pregnancy (Smithels *et al* 1959, 1981). Further studies have demonstrated that vitamin supplementation should be implemented around the time of conception, as no reduction in the incidence is seen for women starting multiple vitamin use after the sixth week of pregnancy (Milunsky *et al* 1989). The Medical Research Council's (MRC) randomised, double-blind, multicentred trial (MRC Vitamin Study Group 1991) examined the effect of folic acid versus multivitamin supplementation or the use of a placebo in women who had previously had an NTD pregnancy. The women were randomly allocated to one of the four supplementation groups. The results showed clear evidence that periconceptional folic acid had a 72 per cent protective effect against the recurrence of an NTD pregnancy. There was no significant effect shown in the other groups. The risk of recurrence was reduced from 3 to 1 per cent.

After this followed the Department of Health (DoH 1992a) recommendation that any woman who had previously had a pregnancy with an NTD should take a periconceptional dose of 5 mg folic acid daily. Strategies developed to ensure that as many of the prepregnancy population as possible benefited from this research. One approach was to target high-risk women: those with a family history of NTDs, those on anticonvulsant therapy or those who lived in poverty with poor diets. However, the occurrence of NTDs and the benefits of folic acid supplementation are not confined to these high-risk groups. Milunsky *et al* (1989) studied a population of well-educated women, in the middle to upper income group, in whom folic acid supplementation was associated with a 70 per cent reduction in the incidence of NTDs. Clearly, targeting only high-risk women is not sufficient.

For the rest of the population of women of reproductive age, an improvement in the diet, particularly an increase in foodstuffs rich in folic acid, should be encouraged prior to pregnancy. A low-dose folic acid supplement is now available for all women periconceptually 'over the counter'. The dose recommended by the Department of Health (1992a) is 400 µg daily until the twelfth week of pregnancy. However, these interventions have the limitation that poorer and less-educated women will be less able to comply. As a way of overcoming this situation, the Department of Health has ensured that some basic foods are fortified with folic acid (DoH 1992a).

The recent evidence relating to folic acid intake and the incidence of NTDs provides a rare opportunity to achieve a major preventive impact on a common and potentially devastating condition by means of a simple and safe nutritional intervention.

■ Pre-existing medical disorders

☐ Diabetes mellitus

Diabetes mellitus has been diagnosed in about half a million people in England and Wales, that is, an estimated 1 per cent of the population, although this may be an underestimate. It has been estimated that for every diagnosed non-insulin dependent diabetic, there is another one undiagnosed. Therefore the prevalence rate is nearer 2 per cent (DoH 1991).

Diabetes depresses the hypothalamic–gonadal axis and would be expected to cause infertility in both men and women (Distiller *et al* 1975). Insulin restores fertility, but before the discovery of insulin, between 95 and 98 per cent of diabetic women were infertile (Gellis & Hsia 1959).

The management of a pregnancy in a woman who has diabetes mellitus is of particular concern for all health care professionals. A poorly managed pregnancy can have serious consequences for both mother and baby. Pederson (1954) first stated that insulin is not teratogenic but glucose is. It is the hyperglycaemia of the mother that stimulates the fetal pancreas to produce insulin. The high fetal insulin levels are responsible for the macrosomia and hypoglycaemia that were once classical in the baby of a diabetic mother.

Before insulin became available in 1922, pregnancy in diabetics was associated with very high fetal loss and a perinatal mortality rate of approximately 60 per cent, but with improved obstetric care and medical management, perinatal mortality rates are now comparable to those of the general population (Matheson & Ethanist 1989). Although these rates have been greatly reduced by advances in insulin therapy, pre-existing diabetes mellitus remains a significant risk to the unborn child. Congenital malformations still account for nearly 50 per cent of deaths amongst infants born to diabetic mothers. Serious malformations are three to four times more likely to occur amongst infants of diabetic mothers than amongst those of non-diabetic mothers (Fuhrman *et al* 1983), and affect 6–9 per cent of all diabetic pregnancies (Miller *et al* 1981). The abnormalities are not only more common, but are also more often severe, multiple and fatal (Steel & Johnstone 1986). These abnormalities include NTDs, microcephaly and heart defects. In the past 10 years, there has been an increasing recognition that the infant and maternal complications associated with diabetes can be prevented by well-maintained prepregnancy and pregnancy glycaemia levels (Steele *et al* 1990).

Thirty to fifty per cent of babies born to diabetic mothers are reported to develop neonatal hypocalcaemia (Tsang *et al* 1981). In a recent study by Demarini *et al* (1994), it was demonstrated that if the maternal blood glucose levels were maintained at less than 6.66 mmol/l

(120 mg/dl) periconceptionally, the rate of neonatal hypocalcaemia in these babies was reduced by 50 per cent of the rate seen in women whose blood glucose levels were maintained at 7.77 mmol/l (140 mg/dl). This evidence adds to the importance of diabetic women maintaining a strict control of their blood sugar prior to pregnancy.

One of the targets of *The health of the nation* (DoH 1991) is to 'achieve a pregnancy outcome in diabetic women that approximates to non-diabetic women'. The specific biological mechanism that causes the congenital malformations seen in pregnancies of diabetic mothers is not clear. However, it is very apparent that the malformations are correlated with the degree of glycaemic control during early pregnancy (Kitzmiller *et al* 1991). If these complications are to be prevented, it is of course necessary to control diabetes well before pregnancy.

One of the first preconception clinics for diabetics was established in 1976 in Edinburgh (Steel *et al* 1982). The aims of the clinic are divided into several distinct areas.

1. The assessment of the woman's fitness for pregnancy. Particular attention is paid to retinopathy, nephropathy, hypertension and ischaemic heart disease, and treatment is initiated as appropriate.

2. Contraceptive advice is given to ensure that pregnancies are planned. The progestogen-only pill is favoured in preference to the combined oral contraceptive pill due to the increased risk of cardio- and cerebrovascular disease in diabetics that is sometimes associated with the combined pill.

3. Infertility is identified and treated.

4. Both the women and their partners are educated about the theory and practice of diabetic care during pregnancy.

5. Optimum diabetic control is monitored using HbA_1 (glycosylated haemoglobin A_1) measurements prior to conception.

6. Healthy lifestyles are encouraged and particular attention is given to discouraging smoking and obesity.

The prepregnancy diabetic clinic has proved invaluable in many areas. It creates close co-operation between the client, her partner, the diabetologist and the obstetrician in the management of the diabetic pregnancy. It also identifies areas of medical concern, including infertility, and has contributed to the decline of unplanned pregnancies, to early diagnosis of the pregnancy and to a more rigid diabetic control from conception (Steel *et al* 1982).

If all known diabetic women were to attend a prepregnancy clinic the Health of the Nation target for pregnancies of diabetic women might then be achieved (Steel *et al* 1982). It would seem logical that this preconception advice should be targeted at diabetic girls at a young age so that they understand the importance of planning their pregnancies and so that appropriate contraceptive methods can be offered. Despite the obvious importance of this intervention, only about one third of women with established diabetes receive preconception care (Janz *et al* 1995). Every visit of a diabetic woman to a health care professional should be regarded as a family planning or preconception opportunity, with consideration of the prevention of the unplanned pregnancies.

☐ **Phenylketonuria**

Phenylketonuria is an inborn error of phenylalanine metabolism. If untreated, it is a major cause of developmental delay. The inheritance is autosomal recessive, and the incidence is 1 in 10–15 000 pregnancies. However, routine neonatal screening for the condition and early dietary treatment have virtually eliminated developmental delay from phenylketonuria (MacCready 1974).

Young women with phenylketonuria who were treated in infancy and childhood are now becoming pregnant. They are, however, at risk of maternal hyperphenylalaninaemia, causing fetal abnormalities and significant developmental delay, if their own phenylalanine levels remain high at conception and during pregnancy. In a prospective study of woman of childbearing age, the efficacy of a phenylalanine-restricted diet in reducing fetal morbidity was evaluated (Platt *et al* 1992). All women were of childbearing age and had blood phenylalanine levels of over 240 µmol/l (4 mg/dl). The phenylalanine-restricted diet was either commenced before pregnancy or during the first, second or third trimesters of pregnancy. The relationship between the fetal abnormalities observed at birth and the average blood phenylalanine levels for all trimesters of pregnancy was evaluated. Optimal fetal outcome appeared to occur when phenylalanine levels of less than 600 µmol/l (10 mg/dl) were achieved by 8–10 weeks gestation and maintained throughout the pregnancy. Ninety per cent of the women with phenylalanine levels of equal to or greater than 1200 µmol/l (20 mg/dl) had microcephalic, intrauterine growth retarded and facially dysmorphic babies.

It is evident from this work that preconception counselling is essential for women with phenylketonuria in order to reduce the risk of infant morbidity.

☐ **Epilepsy**

An increased incidence of congenital abnormalities (including dysmorphic facial appearance, NTDs and multiple malformations) has been demonstrated in offspring born to both treated and untreated mothers with epilepsy (Dalessio 1985; Rosa 1991). The use of antiepileptic drugs during pregnancy is associated with a further increased risk of congenital malformations due to their teratogenic effect (Omtzigt *et al* 1992). In a prospective study of 96 pregnant women exposed to valproic acid at conception and during pregnancy, the overall incidence of abnormalities was 8.3 per cent and the incidence of spina bifida 6.3 per cent (Omtzigt *et al* 1992).

Although the precise biochemical mechanism for the teratogenic effects of valproic acid and other antiepileptic drugs is unknown, studies suggest that the altered folate metabolism and/or interference with folate metabolism may be partly responsible (Dansky *et al* 1992).

Medical advice should be sought by women with epilepsy prior to pregnancy to try to minimise the effect of the anticonvulsant therapy on the fetus. Folic acid supplementation should be commenced periconceptionally (Dansky *et al* 1992). If valproic acid cannot be avoided during pregnancy, dose reduction should be considered (Omtzigt *et al* 1992).

■ Smoking

A detailed discussion of the recent research relating to smoking in pregnancy is beyond the scope of this chapter: a brief résumé only is given here. The reader is referred to Plant (1990) and Chapter 5 in this volume.

Smoking in pregnancy is associated with low birthweight babies and a 28 per cent increase in perinatal mortality (DoH 1991). Cliver *et al* (1995) showed that neonates born to mothers who reported smoking in the first trimester of pregnancy had an overall 4% reduction in birthweight compared with babies of non-smoking mothers. Babies born to mothers who continued to smoke throughout the pregnancy had a reduction in their birthweight of 5.9 per cent, but there was only a 1.7 per cent reduction for babies born to mothers who stopped smoking after the first trimester. Stopping smoking was significantly associated with increases in birthweight and fetal measurements, whereas reducing the number of cigarettes smoked in the first trimester was not.

Associations have also been demonstrated between smoking and infertility, menstrual disorders, spontaneous abortions, ectopic pregnancies, placental irregularities, and infant and childhood morbidity (Cefalo & Moos 1988).

In an attempt to help the client stop smoking, the midwife should not just be concerned with the risks caused to the fetus, but should be aware of the difficulties that the client will experience in stopping smoking, and should be reassuring and encouraging throughout. Follow-up support and advice should always be provided during the maintenance programme (Prochaska & Diclemente 1986).

■ Alcohol

A detailed discussion of the recent research literature relating to alcohol in pregnancy is outside the scope of this chapter, and the reader is referred to Plant (1990) and Chapter 5 in this volume.

The consequences of very high alcohol levels in pregnancy are now well known. Babies born to women with a chronic alcohol problem have particular congenital anomalies that are collectively known as the 'fetal alcohol syndrome' (Jones *et al* 1973); these include dysmorphic facial features, intrauterine growth retardation and developmental delay. Alcohol consumption around the time of conception and during pregnancy is also associated with spontaneous abortions and low birthweight babies (Plant 1987). Unfortunately, heavy drinkers (more than 14 drinks per week) may be less likely than moderate drinkers to recognise the influence of alcohol in pregnancy (Lelong *et al* 1995).

Fetal alcohol syndrome is the severe end of the spectrum of alcohol consumption in pregnancy, but a lesser daily consumption of three units of alcohol throughout pregnancy has been linked to behavioural disorders in children and there is also an average decrease in their I.Q. by 5–7 points (Larroque *et al* 1992). There is no evidence, however, of an increased risk to the child when the consumption is around one or two units once or twice a week (Mills *et al* 1986; Plant 1987; Larroque *et al* 1992).

In the preconception counselling session, midwives can play an important part in informing women of the potential hazards of alcohol consumption during pregnancy, and helping them to modify their behaviour prior to pregnancy and sustain that modification throughout the pregnancy, by continual support. The midwife should be able to identify, through careful interviewing, women with an alcohol problem and refer them to specialised services for intervention before pregnancy. Again this presents a problem, as the dependent or heavy drinker frequently denies that there is a dependency problem and would perhaps be less likely to present for preconception advice than would others.

■ Family planning

While taking a contraceptive history, it is appropriate to discuss the client's future reproductive planning. It is at this time that it would seem logical to introduce the concept of preconception care. Advice should be given to the client who is planning a pregnancy to attend the family planning clinic, especially if she is either taking the oral contraceptive pill or has an intrauterine contraceptive device (IUCD) fitted.

☐ **The oral contraceptive pill**

Oral contraception includes both the combined pill (oestrogen and pro-
gestogen pill) and the progestogen-only pill (the mini pill). Oestrogen
acts by suppressing the secretions of the gonadotrophins and thus
inhibiting ovulation. An atrophic endometrium is produced by both pro-
gestogen and oestrogen, making it unreceptive to implantation. The cervical mucus also becomes tenacious, impairing the passage of sperm
(Guillebaud 1993).

The combined and progestogen-only pill should be discontinued for
at least one month before conception (Belfield 1993). This will increase
the opportunity for a regular ovulatory and menstrual cycle to be
resumed as oestrogen and progesterone levels and the other physiological
changes return to normal. It will, in addition, aid in the identification of
ovulation so that the couple can accurately time their fertile period, and
will increase the accuracy of dating the pregnancy. Mineral and vitamin
(especially folate) metabolism will also have a chance to return to normal
(Guillebaud 1993) There is, however, no good evidence to conclude that
conception immediately following the discontinuation of oral contracep-
tives has any negative influence on pregnancy outcome.

☐ **The intrauterine contraceptive device (IUCD)**

In situ, the IUCD produces endometrial changes incompatible with
implantation and also alters uterine and tubal fluids so that they impair
the viability of the gamete (Drife 1993). The copper element of the
device produces a foreign-body reaction in the endometrium. The IUCD
must be removed before pregnancy, and fertility is unimpaired following
its removal.

■ **Screening for health**

☐ **Blood tests**

Rubella vaccination
As rubella has a teratogenic effect on the fetus, it is important that any
woman who is considering a pregnancy should have her rubella immunity checked prior to conception. If a woman is found to be non-
immune, vaccination can then be given. However, the couple should be
advised not to conceive for a month following the vaccination, and effective contraception should be taken in the meantime (DoH 1992b). The
immunity status should then be rechecked after this time.

Haemoglobin
The haemoglobin level should be checked, and the underlying cause for any anaemia should be corrected prior to a pregnancy.

Haemoglobinopathies: sickle cell disease and thalassaemias
During the preconception consultation, it is extremely important to ask the couple the country of their parental origin to ascertain the likelihood of their being carriers of either of these two haemoglobinopathies. Sickle cell disease results from a glutamic acid to valine mutation in the beta globin chain. The carrier frequency approaches 1 in 8 in some parts of Africa. The condition is inherited in an autosomal recessive manner, so only couples who are both carriers will be at risk of having affected children.

The thalassaemias are characterised by a failure of globin chain synthesis. They are also autosomal recessively inherited conditions. Beta thalassaemia major is an important cause of perinatal death in some parts of the Mediterranean, the Middle East and Asia. In South-East Asia, alpha thalassaemia contributes to a number of intrauterine and neonatal deaths.

Anyone a risk of being a carrier for the thalassaemia or sickle cell trait should be given advice concerning carrier screening prior to pregnancy.

Screening for HIV antibodies
This should be offered to the high-risk populations so that appropriate contraception can be employed, preventing unwanted pregnancies and providing protection for the partner. It is essential that a pre- and post-test counselling service is available. For further information on HIV and pregnancy, the reader is referred to Roth (1995).

□ **Urinalysis**

The urine should be screened for proteinuria to exclude a chronic renal disease, and glycosuria to exclude undiagnosed diabetes mellitus. In both instances, it is essential that abnormal results are investigated fully prior to a pregnancy to ensure that the client is in an optimum state of health before conception.

■ **Genetic counselling**

Genetic counselling has been defined as 'the process by which patients or their relatives at risk of a disorder that may be hereditary are advised of the consequences of the disorder, the probability of developing or transmitting it and the ways in which it may be prevented, avoided or ameliorated' (Harper 1981: 3). Genetic counselling is informative, supportive and enabling (Clarke 1990), and should be non-directive when possible (Clarke 1991). In order to have any impact upon the occurrence of disorders with an inherited element, preconception care must be primarily concerned with the recognition of couples or individuals who are at risk of having offspring with specific disorders. When at-risk individuals are identified, they may then be referred to a clinical genetics department, where counselling and information concerning their risk and reproductive options is available.

During the past decade, the demand for genetic counselling has steadily increased. The main reasons for this increase are:

- A growing public interest in the genetic background of disease;

- The introduction of DNA technology, making it possible to trace the inheritance of important disease genes through families;

- The availability of prenatal screening programmes for fetal abnormalities.

DNA technology has provided genetic 'handles' for an ever-increasing number of diseases, and for some, prenatal diagnosis is now available. Before DNA technology, a diagnosis of a predisposition to genetic disease was based on family history. However, it is now possible, before the onset of symptoms, to determine with some degree of accuracy whether an individual is a carrier or is likely to develop any one of numerous diseases. Some disease genes have now been cloned, and definitive presymptomatic carrier testing is now available for some conditions, for example myotonic dystrophy (Fu *et al* 1992) and Huntington's disease (Huntington's disease Collaborative Group 1993). It is now possible to determine whether someone is a carrier of a recessively inherited condition (for example cystic fibrosis, Rommens *et al* 1989) or an X-linked condition (for example fragile X mental retardation, Oberle *et al* 1991; or Duchenne muscular dystrophy, Koenig *et al* 1987).

The optimum time to give genetic information to a client is before a pregnancy, and the aim of any midwife in a preconception clinic should be to take a thorough family history. Questions should include the following.

- Is there any medical condition in either the client's or the partner's family that they think could be inherited?

- Is there a family history of unexplained stillbirths, infant deaths or recurrent miscarriages?

- Is there anyone in either family with learning difficulties?

- Is there a family history of cystic fibrosis?

- Is there a family history of muscular dystrophy?

- Are the couple related to each other?

If the answer to any of these questions is yes, advice should be sought from the local clinical genetics service. The client can if necessary then be referred. Further family details and confirmation of the diagnosis will be obtained prior to the genetic clinic appointment. Investigations may include chromosomal and DNA analysis if appropriate.

Reproductive options will be discussed in the light of the risk of recurrence for the client. The availability and acceptability of prenatal diagnosis (amniocentesis, chorionic villus sampling and detailed ultrasound scanning; Whelton 1993) should be discussed with the client. The provision of detailed information for clients prior to pregnancy enables them to make an informed decision about their reproductive future.

Genetic counselling is important not only for those with an increased risk of a genetic condition, but also for those who are not at an increased risk of a genetic condition but who have their own anxieties about possible risks. Explanation given in the preconception period may allow parents to be less anxious during pregnancy.

■ Recommendations for clinical practice in the light of currently available evidence

1. The midwife should recognise that all women of childbearing age who present themselves in primary health care settings, family planning clinics and other women's health care settings are candidates for preconception care.

2. All midwives should be aware of the findings of the Medical Research Council's multivitamin trial (MRC Vitamin Study Group 1991) and the Department of Health's recommendations concerning folic acid supplementation (DoH 1992a).

3. Midwives should make prompt referrals to the clinical genetics unit when a potential genetic problem is identified, so that time is allowed to investigate the concern fully and to instigate appropriate tests prior to pregnancy.

4. Midwives involved in health promotion programmes should be sensitive and encouraging in realising the potential difficulties that clients can experience when withdrawing from nicotine or alcohol.

5. When an area of concern has been identified by the client or the midwife, every effort should be made to provide the highest quality of service and information to the client at this very vulnerable time in her life.

6. Preconception care should be multidisciplinary, and referrals to other

health care professionals should be made in order that the client can make an informed choice about her reproductive future based on accurate and up to date information.

■ Lay support groups

Foresight is an association for the promotion of preconception care. It can be contacted via the address given at the end of the chapter.

■ Practice check

- Do you currently provide preconception advice within your practice?

- What facilities are offered in your workplace to provide preconception advice?

- Does the local health promotion department have literature available (for example leaflets, videos and posters) that you can use to enhance your practice area and advertise that preconception advice is available?

- Where are the local family planning clinics held and do they offer preconception clinics?

- Where is the local clinical genetics service? How is a referral made to the service? Can it be used as a resource centre?

- If you wanted to become involved in the setting up of a preconception clinic, whom would you contact within your local area? What could you do within your present resources and available funds to promote health prior to conception?

- Are there 'well person' clinics in your area?

- Does your area have a local phone-in 'health line' giving advice on a range of health issues, and if so, is preconception advice available?

- How do your local perinatal, neonatal and maternal mortality rates compare with the national average and are they decreasing in line with the Health of the Nation targets?

- Have you read any books or articles or attended any study sessions on preconception care?

- Do you know how to contact Foresight?

■ References

Abrams BF, Laros RK 1986 Pre pregnancy weight, weight gain and birth weight. American Journal of Obstetrics and Gynecology   154: 503–9

Abrams BF, Neuman V 1989 Maternal weight gain and pre-term delivery. Obstetrics and Gynecology   74: 377–83

Adams MM, Bruce FC, Shulman HB, Kendrick JS, Brogan DJ and the PRAMS Working Group 1993 Pregnancy planning and pre-conception counselling. Obstetrics and Gynecology   82 (6): 955–9

Belfield T 1993 FPA contraceptive handbook. Family Planning Association, London, Ch 4, p32–54

Cefalo RC, Moos MK 1988 Preconceptional health promotion: a practical guide. Aspen, Rockville, MD

Clarke A 1990 Genetics, ethics and audit. Lancet   335: 1145–7

Clarke A 1991 Is non-directive genetic counselling possible? Lancet   338: 998–1001

Cliver SP, Goldenberg RL, Cutter GR, Hoffman HJ, Davis RO, Nelson KG 1995 The effect of cigarette smoking on neonatal anthropometric measurements. Obstetrics and Gynaecology   85(4): 625–30

Copper RL, DuBard MB, Goldenberg RL, Oweis AI 1995 The relationship of maternal attitude toward weight gain during pregnancy and low birth weight. Obstetrics and Gynecology   85(4): 591–5

Dalessio DJ 1985 Current concepts: seizure disorders and pregnancy. New England Journal of Medicine   312: 559–63

Dansky LV, Rosenblatt DS, Andermann E 1992 Mechanisms of teratogenesis: folic acid and antiepileptic therapy. Neurology   42(supplement 5): 32–42

Demarini S, Mimouni F, Tsang RC, Khoury J, Hertzberg V 1994 Impact of metabolic control of diabetes during pregnancy on neonatal hypocalcemia: a randomized study. Obstetrics and Gynecology   83(6): 918–22

Department of Health 1991 The health of the nation. HMSO, London

Department of Health 1992a Folic acid and the preventation of neural tube defects: report from an Expert Advisory Group. Health Publications, Heywood

Department of Health 1992b Immunisation against infectious disease. HMSO, London

Distiller LA, Sagel J, Morley JE, Joffe BI, Seftel HC 1975 Pituitary responsiveness to luteinizing-hormone releasing hormone in insulin-dependent diabetes mellitus. Diabetes   24: 378–80

Drife JO 1993 Intrauterine contraceptive devices. In: Loudon N (ed.) Handbook of family planning. Churchill Livingstone, Edinburgh, Ch 7, p161–87

Frisch RE, McArthur JW 1974 Menstrual cycles: fatness as a determinant of minimum weight for height necessary for their maintenance or onset. Science 185: 949–51

Fu VH, Pizzuti A, Fenwick RJ Jr 1992 An unstable triplet repeat in a gene related to myotonic dystrophy. Science   255: 1256–8

Fuhrman K, Reiher H, Semmler K 1983 Prevention of congenital malformations in infants of insulin-dependent diabetic mothers. Diabetic Care   6: 219–23

Gellis SS, Hsia Y-YD 1959 The infant of the diabetic mother. American Journal of Diseases of Children   97: 1–41

Guillebaud J 1993 Combined oral contraceptive pills. In: Loudon N (ed.)

Handbook of family planning. Churchill Livingstone, Edinburgh, Ch 4, p63–123

Haller E 1992 Eating disorders – a review and update. Western Journal of Medicine 157(6): 658–62

Harper PS 1981 Practical genetic counselling. Butterworth-Heinemann, Cambridge

Huntington's disease Collaborative Research Group 1993 A novel gene containing a triuncleotide repeat that is expanded and unstable of Huntington disease chromosomes. Cell 72: 971–83

Jack BW, Culpepper L 1990 Preconception care. Risk reduction and health promotion in preparation for pregnancy. Journal of the American Medical Association 264: 1147–9

Jack BW, Culpepper L 1991 Preconception care. Journal of Family Practice 32(3): 306–12

Janz NK, Herman WH, Becker MP, Charronprochownik D, Shayna VL, Lesnick TG, Jacober SJ, Fachnie JD, Kruger DF, Sanfield JA, Rosenblatt SI, Lorenz RP 1995 Diabetes and pregnancy – factors associated with seeking pre-conception care. Diabetes Care 18(2): 157–65

Jones KL, Smith DW, Ulleland CN, Streissguth AP 1973 Pattern of malformation in offspring of chronic alcoholic mothers. Lancet i: 1267–71

Kitzmiller JL, Gavin LA, Gin GD, Jovanovic-Peterson L, Main EK, Zigrang WD 1991 Preconception care of diabetes: glycemic control prevents congenital malformations. Journal of the American Medical Association 265: 731–6

Koenig M, Hoffman EP, Bertelson CJ 1987 Complete cloning of the Duchenne muscular dystrophy (DMD) cDNA. Cell 50: 509–17

Larroque B, Kaminiski, Dehaene P 1992 Maternal alcohol consumption during pregnancy and child development at 4 years. Journal of Perinatal Medicine 20 (supplement 1)

Lelong N, Kaminski M, Chwalow J, Bean K, Subtil D 1995 Attitudes and behaviour of pregnant women and health professionals towards alcohol and tobacco consumption. Patient Education and Counselling 25: 39–49

MacCready RA 1974 Admissions of phenylketonuric patients to residential institutions before and after screening programmes of the newborn infant. Journal of Paediatrics 85: 383–5

Matheson D, Ethanist J 1989 Diabetes and pregnancy: need and use of intensive therapy. Diabetes Education 15: 242–8

Miller E, Hare JW, Cloherty J P 1981 Elevated maternal haemoglobin a1c in early pregnancy and major congenital anomalies in infants of diabetic mothers. New England Journal of Medicine 304:1331–4

Mills JL, Graubard BI, Harley EE, Rhoads GG, Berendes HW 1986 Maternal alcohol consumption and birth weight. How much drinking during pregnancy is safe? Journal of the American Medical Association 252: 1875–9

Milunsky A, Jick H, Jick S, Bruell CL, MacLaughlin DS, Rothman KJ, Willett W 1989 Multivitamin/folic acid supplementation in early pregnancy reduces the prevalence of neural tube defects. Journal of the American Medical Association 262: 2847–52

Montgomery E 1993 Iron and vitamin supplementation during pregnancy. In Alexander J, Levy V, Roch S (eds) Midwifery practice: a research-based approach. Macmillan, Basingstoke, Ch 2, p20–34

MRC Vitamin Study Group 1991 Prevention of neural tube defects: results of the Medical Research Council Vitamin Study. Lancet   338: 131–7

Oberle I, Rousseau F, Heitz D 1991 Instability of a 550 basic pair DNA segment and abnormal methylation in fragile X syndrome. Science   252: 1097–102

Omtzigt JGC, Los FJ, Grobee DE, Pijpers L, Jahoda MGJ 1992 The risk of spina bifida aperta after first trimester exposure to valporate in prenatal cohort. Neurology   42 (supplement 5): 119–25

Pederson J 1954 Weight and length at birth of infants of diabetic mothers. Acta Endocrinologica   16: 330–41

Plant ML 1987 Women drinking and pregnancy. Tavistock, London

Plant ML 1990 Maternal alcohol and tobacco use during pregnancy. In Alexander J, Levy V, Roch S (eds) Antenatal care: a research-based approach. Macmillan, Basingstoke, Ch 5, p73–87

Platt LD, Koch R, Azen C, Hanley W, Levy H, Matalon R, Rouse B, de la Cruz F, Walla C 1992 Maternal phenylketonuria collaborative, obstetric aspects and outcome: the first 6 years. American Journal of Obstetrics and Gynecology 166(4): 1151–60

Prochaska JO, Diclemente C 1986 Towards a comprehensive model of change. In Miller WR, Heather N (eds) Treating addictive behaviours: processes of change. Plenum Press, New York, p3–27

Rommens JM, Ianuzzi MC, Kerem B 1989 Identification of the cystic fibrosis gene: chromosome walking and jumping. Science   245: 1059–65

Rosa FW 1991 Spina bifida in infants of women treated with carbamazepine during pregnancy. New England Journal of Medicine   324: 674–7

Roth C 1995 HIV and pregnancy. In Alexander J, Levy V, Roch S (eds) Aspects of midwifery practice: a research-based approach. Macmillan, Basingstoke, Ch 6, p109–31

Smithells RW, Sheppard S, Schorah CJ 1959 Vitamin levels and neural tube defects. Archives of Disease in Childhood   51: 944–50

Smithells R W, Sheppard S, Schorah CJ 1981 Apparent prevention of neural tube defects by perinconceptional vitamin supplementation. Archives of Disease in Childhood   56: 911–18

Spedding S, Wilson J, Wright S, Jackson A 1995 Nutrition for pregnancy and lactation. In Alexander J, Levy W, Roch S (eds) Aspects of midwifery practice: a research-based approach. Macmillan, Basingstoke, Ch 1, p 1–23

Steel JM, Johnstone FD 1986 Prepregnancy management of the diabetic. In Chamberlain G, Lumley L (eds) Pregnancy care: a manual for practice. John Wiley & Sons, London, p165–182

Steel J M, Johnstone F D, Smith A F, Duncun L J P 1982 Five years experience of a 'prepregnancy' clinic for insulin dependent diabetics. British Medical Journal 285: 353–6

Steel JM, Johnstone FD, Hepurn DA, Smith AF 1990 Can pre-pregnancy care of diabetic women reduce the risk of abnormal babies? British Medical Journal 301: 1070–4

Tsang RC, Ballard J, Braun C 1981 The infants of diabetic mothers: today and tomorrow. Clinical Obstetrics and Gynecology   24: 125–47

Warren MP 1980 The effects of exercise on pubertal progression and reproductive functioning girls. Journal of Clinical Endocrinology and Metabolism   51: 1150–7

Whelton J 1993 Fetal medicine. In Alexander J, Levy V, Roch S (eds) Midwifery
     practice: a research-based approach. Macmillan, Basingstoke, Ch 4, p55–73
Wynn M, Wynn A 1981 Historical associations of congenital malformations.
     International Journal of Environmental Studies   71: 7–12

■ Suggested further reading

Barnes B, Bradley SG 1994 Planning for a healthy baby: essential preparation for
     pregnancy. Vermilion, London
Chamberlain G, Lumley J 1986 Prepregnancy care: a manual for practice. John
     Wiley & Sons, Chichester
Harper PS 1993 Practical genetic counselling, 4th edn. Butterworth–Heinemann,
     Cambridge
Robarts PJ 1990 Preparing for pregnancy. Faber & Faber, London
Wynn M, Wynn A 1991 The case for preconception care of men and women. AB
     Academic, Bicester

■ Useful addresses

Association for the Improvement of Maternity Services (AIMS)
Goose Green Barn
Much Hoole
Preston
Lancs PR4 4TD

Foresight
28 The Paddock
Godalming
Surrey GU7 1XD

Support Around Termination for Abnormality (SAFTA)
29–30 Soho Square
London W1V 6JB

Chapter 3

Antenatal risk assessment

Jennifer Wilson

Few women in the West now fear for their lives as they approach child-birth (Enkin 1994), and, with the perinatal mortality rate in England and Wales currently being less than nine per thousand (OPCS 1994), most pregnant women will give birth to a live baby. It might appear that the risks associated with pregnancy are falling, but it also seems that the subject of antenatal risk assessment is attracting increasing interest (James & Stirrat 1988). This is perhaps most evident in the assessment of genetic risk, where the results of antenatal screening tests are increasingly precise (Donnai 1988). However, midwives have a particular role in relation to the main purpose of risk assessment, that is, to assist each pregnant woman to become a healthy mother of a healthy baby.

■ **It is assumed that you are already aware of the following:**

- The principles of good antenatal care.

■ **Why assess risk?**

When the Cranbrook Committee of 1959 (Ministry of Health 1959) suggested how women with high-risk pregnancies could be identified, the purpose was to encourage these women to have their babies in hospital, then considered to be the safest place for giving birth (Tew 1990). Today, one of the main purposes of risk assessment continues to be to assist decision making about the most appropriate care for pregnant women, including the place, frequency and provider of that care. Midwives are particularly involved in this.

There are four main reasons why risk assessment is increasingly relevant for midwives.

First, as described in Chapter 1 of this volume, the number of maternity care schemes available in Britain, often involving teams of midwives, units led by midwives and midwifery group practices, has recently and rapidly increased. Options of how and where to give birth are also likely to increase, with, for example, home birth services being developed in response to government recommendations (DoH 1993; Scottish Office Home and Health Department 1993) and water births arousing more interest (Diamond 1994). Advancing technology has also increased the sophistication and number of tests available to monitor a pregnancy (Whelton 1993). Such changes mean that pregnant women now face more decisions than ever before.

Second, the midwife, being the professional who usually takes a woman's booking history and who is often the main, and likely in the future to be the only, provider of maternity care for many women, has particular responsibilities for risk assessment. Her clinical responsibility to the expectant mother is to recognise potential risks and to respond appropriately to minimise them. She also has a professional responsibility to adhere to the Midwives' Rules (UKCC 1993). It may be naive to assume that the presence of a risk factor (a characteristic observed as being associated with an abnormality: US Department of Health and Human Services 1989; Aikins Murphy 1994) always precedes the development of that abnormality, which can then be averted or minimised by intervention or precautionary action. Rarely do threatened complications arise, and often they are unpreventable (Hall 1990). However, while definitions of normality vary (Downe 1994), the Midwives' Rules (p20) state that the detection of a 'deviation from the norm' requires the assistance of a registered medical practitioner. Thus, for a midwife to ignore a recognised risk factor would be foolhardy.

Third, the importance of involving the expectant mother in decisions about her maternity care, including whom she should see, has recently been emphasized in *Changing childbirth*, the report of the Expert Maternity Group (DoH 1993). Amongst all concerned, it is probably the mother who has the greatest interest in her own and her baby's well-being, but also she who often has the least knowledge. For a woman to make sensible and appropriate choices regarding her care – the personnel involved, the investigations and tests she undergoes, the treatment she receives and where and how she has her baby – she needs to be able to understand and weigh up the risks involved for her personally (Page 1994). It is likely to be her midwife, probably the main provider of her maternity care, to whom she turns for the explanations, advice and support she needs. Thus a midwife needs sufficient knowledge not only to recognise risk factors so that she can make appropriate referrals, but also to understand and be able to explain why they are considered risky.

Finally, litigation against providers of maternity care is increasing, possibly contributing to the growing interest in risk assessment (Enkin

1994). It cost the NHS in the UK £150 million in 1994 (Steer 1994). Over 75 per cent of American obstetricians have now had at least one claim made against them (American College of Obstetricians and Gynecologists 1992). Practising midwives are not immune from this threat. In attempts to improve care and thus reduce the likelihood of legal action, some maternity units in the UK have recently appointed someone (often a midwife) with a job title such as 'Risk Manager' with this specifically in mind (O'Connor, pers comm 1995). It is perhaps ironic that one of the early uses of the word 'risk' in the English language in the 19th century was in association with insurance (Moore 1983).

Risk assessment is also of interest to epidemiologists at local, national and international levels, contributing, for example, to the discussion about whether the new maternity care schemes being introduced in Britain are likely to achieve the high levels of safety for mother and baby that are now expected (Cole & McIlwaine 1994). Cole and McIlwaine (1994) have demonstrated how, by using the presence or absence of certain risk factors to divide women into risk categories, predictions can be made about the effects of encouraging low-risk women to have their babies at home or in a GP or midwifery unit. Defining populations of pregnant women by their risk status in this way has been used for several epidemiological studies and is becoming the basis for many public health strategies (Alexander & Keirse 1989). The World Health Organization (WHO) sees this 'risk approach' as a policy and managerial tool with great potential to guide future health care planners in resource allocation (Alexander & Keirse 1989) and thus to redress inequalities in maternal and child health around the world (Backett *et al* 1984).

Indeed, risk assessment may already have contributed to reductions, at least in the West, in maternal and perinatal mortality rates (Mendez-Bauer *et al* 1994). While the precise causes of many complications of pregnancy remain elusive, researching and identifying various socioeconomic, medical, gynaecological and obstetric risk factors has shown how risks can be reduced. Thus, risk assessment and the identification of risk factors can also be helpful to medical and midwifery educators, helping students to understand the prognosis of pregnancy (Alexander & Kerise 1989).

■ Assessing risk – the problems

There is a general assumption that high-risk pregnancies can be identified (Chard *et al* 1994). However, complications of pregnancy or labour that do arise often occur unexpectedly in those considered to be of low risk (Scherger 1988). Equally, all midwives will know of women with complicated medical or obstetric histories who, apparently against all the odds, have sailed through pregnancy and labour.

A particular problem in risk assessment for midwives and mothers is that it is often difficult to define the problem they are hoping to avoid; 'Risk of what?' may be a difficult question for midwives and mothers to answer. Although techniques have been developed for evaluating, for example, the risk of premature labour or fetal death (see Alexander & Keirse 1989), it is generally something as vague as 'things going wrong' that midwives are trying to avoid.

Furthermore, the phrase 'things going wrong' is open to personal interpretation. For example, a planned home birth that becomes an emergency caesarean section may perhaps be more disappointing for the midwife than for the mother, delighted with her healthy newborn. Pregnant women may also differ from each other in their perceptions of risk. Oakley (1992) cites two women as an example of this, one with two previous low birthweight (LBW) children, the other with only one. In their subsequent pregnancies, the first considered herself perfectly normal, while the latter felt she was beset with potential problems. Risk assessment is thus very subjective, depending on one's understanding of risk, experience and expectations (James & Stirrat 1988; Handwerker 1994).

In practice, most midwives and obstetricians have their own ideas of what constitutes a risky pregnancy. Few would now agree with the belief of Hippocrates' day that a 'damp mild winter ... followed by a dry spring' was likely to lead to miscarriage (Lloyd 1983: 214). Many would include some of the factors listed in Table 3.1 amongst those they consider to be risky. Some, like Reynolds *et al* (1988), would doubt whether the criteria of 1967, based on the Cranbrook Committee's recommendations of 1959 (Ministry of Health 1959), are still adequate as the basis on which women are booked for GP care. These criteria were that women should have uncompromised medical and obstetric histories, nulliparae should be taller than 152 cm and less than 30 years of age, and multiparae should be less than 35 years old and of parity less than four.

However, the debate continues over which factors really are risky and how each should be defined. For example, is a 'redhead' really more inclined to haemorrhage than other women, and exactly how old is 'elderly' – 35, 37 or 40 years? Clinicians have been trying to reach agreement about these and similar questions for centuries. This debate has resulted in a variety of conditions and situations being considered worthy of inclusion on lists of risk factors produced by, and used in, some maternity units. The author's own survey in 1995 of seven maternity units known to her in southern England revealed eight markedly different lists in use there (Table 3.1). (The survey was conducted for this chapter and is not published elsewhere.)

Even if all who may be involved in a woman's maternity care agree on the factors they judge to be risky, they must also consider what should be done in the event of one or more of these factors being present. This question is particularly pertinent for the midwife, who is likely to

Table 3.1 Simplified lists of risk factors used by seven maternity units known to the author in southern England and in the Netherlands

	A	B	C	D	E	F	G		Netherlands
Type of unit	Consultant unit	Consultant unit	Consultant unit	Consultant unit	Midwifery unit	Consultant unit	Consultant unit		
Purpose of list	Increased frequency of antenatal visits	Obstetric led care in conjunction with midwifery care	Medical consultation	Referal to obstetric consultant, day assessment unit or fetal assessment unit	Admission/delivery in consultant unit	Referal to consultant	(a) Referal to consultant	(b) Guide to possible reasons for referal to another agency	Specialist obstetric care
Factors found at booking									
Parity	*								*
'Old' age	*	*		*	*	*	*	*	*
Youth	*			*	*	*	*	*	
Short stature	*								
Overweight	*	*		*	*	*	*	*	
Underweight	*							*	
Smoking	*							*	
Alcohol abuse	*							*	
Drug abuse	*			*	*	*	*	*	
Social problems	*							*	
Not fluent in English		*						*	
Cot death				*	*				
Late booking/ no antenatal care			*					*	
At school			*						
Separated/unsupported			*					*	
Economic problems			*					*	
Domestic violence			*					*	
Physical/sexual abuse			*					*	
Previous 'at risk'		*	*					*	
Professional concern								*	
Medical history									
Diabetes	*	*	*	*	*	*	*		*
Cardiac disease	*	*	*	*	*	*	*		*
Renal disease		*	*	*		*	*		
Hypertension	*	*	*	*	*	*	*		
Embolism/thrombosis		*	*			*			
Chest disease		*	*	*		*			
Central nervous system disorders		*		*		*			*
Endocrine disorders		*		*		*			
Rhesus disease/antibodies	*	*		*			*		*

Autoimmune disease
Hepatitis B
HIV
Psychiatric history
Blood disease
Haemoglobinopathies
Tuberculosis
Kyphoscoliosis
Cystic fibrosis
Hereditary condition
in family
Immune thrombocytopenia
purpura
Systemic lupus
erythematosus
Rheumatoid arthritis
Liver problems
Crohn's disease/
ulcerative colitis
Toxoplasmosis
Other

Gynaecological history
Recent infertility
Reproductive tract
anomaly
Hysterotomy/myomectomy
Pelvic floor repair
Abortions/miscarriages
Uncertain last menstrual
period
Intrauterine contraceptive
device *in situ*
Other

Obstetric history
Cervical suture
Hypertensive disorders
Preterm delivery
Small baby
Large baby
Proven/suspected
cephalopelvic
disproportion
Precipitate labour
Long labour and/or
difficult vaginal delivery

Table 3.1 Continued

	A	B	C	D	E	F	G (a)	G (b)	Netherlands
Type of unit	Consultant unit	Consultant unit	Consultant unit	Consultant unit	Midwifery unit	Consultant unit	Consultant unit	Consultant unit	
Purpose of list	Increased frequency of antenatal visits	Obstetric led care in conjunction with midwifery care	Medical consultation	Referal to obstetric consultant, day assessment unit or fetal assessment unit	Admission/delivery in consultant unit	Referal to consultant	Referal to consultant	Guide to possible reasons for referral to another agency	Specialist obstetric care
Placental abruption	*								
Caesarean section		*		*	*		*		*
Severe perineal tear		*	*	*	*	*	*		*
Postpartum haemorrhage	*	*				*			*
Retained placenta	*								
Uterine rupture			*						*
Stillbirth/neonatal death	*	*	*	*	*	*	*	*	*
Abnormal/handicapped baby	*	*	*	*	*		*		*
Postnatal depression	*								
Other									
Factors found during pregnancy or labour									
Ectopic pregnancy	*		*			*	*		
Trophoblastic disease			*			*	*		
Abnormal antibodies	*	*	*	*		*	*		
Abnormal screening tests		*		*		*	*		
Anaemia	*		*			*			
Jaundice									
Albuminuria alone									
Rubella contact									
Hyperemesis gravidarum									
Abnormal glucose tolerance test				*					
Abnormal ultrasound scan	*		*		*				
Urinary tract/vaginal infection	* *		*		*				
Proteinuria	* *	*							
Hypertensive disorders, including eclampsia	* *	*	*	*	* * *	* *	* *		*
Polyhydramnios									
Oligohydramnios									

Intrauterine growth
  retardation
Vaginal bleeding
Premature labour/
  rupture of membranes
Multiple pregnancy
Reduced fetal movements
Poor weight gain
Large for dates
Abnormal antenatal
  cardiotocograph/fetal
  heart rate
Malpresentation/unstable
  lie nearing term
Primigravida with
  'high head' at term
Term spontaneous rupture
  of membranes
Prolonged pregnancy
Needing induction of
  labour
Poor progress in labour
Requesting epidural
Fetal distress/meconium-
  stained liquor
Active herpes
Maternal concern re
  previous delivery
Other

Many of the risk factors were more precisely defined in the original lists.

be the first to identify risk factors in the majority of women. Should she, for example, recommend to every woman with a history of a forceps delivery that she sees an obstetrician antenatally? Such a woman is less likely to require an obstetrician's attention before delivery than is one with a classical caesarean scar on her uterus. The relative contribution of different factors to risk must be considered. What about the woman with none of the given risk factors, but about whom the midwife feels uneasy? Every midwife must use her discretion, clinical judgement and perhaps intuition in assessing risk, regardless of the clarity of the policies and procedures of the unit within which she works or the length of her list of risk factors, which can never be exhaustive. Her decisions will inevitably depend in part on the local situation. It would be quite understandable for a midwife to vary the advice she gives, or the action she recommends, depending on whether a woman is planning to give birth in an isolated situation or within a consultant unit.

Antenatal risk assessment must be an ongoing process. The booking appointment is certainly of great importance as this is usually the midwife's first opportunity to identify potential problems (Lilford *et al* 1992), but a pregnant woman's risk status may change at any time, sometimes rapidly, during pregnancy and labour, with, for example, rising blood pressure. Bearing in mind that many adverse events of the post-natal period, such as postpartum haemorrhage or eclampsia, may be the result of a worsening condition that existed before delivery, antenatal risk assessment must be maintained from before conception (where possible) (Andolsek 1993) right through to the completion of labour.

■ Identifying high-risk pregnancies

□ How is it done?

Despite the difficulties, and particularly in view of the increasing threat of litigation, there seems to be a need for objective methods of assessing risk in antenatal women. In its most simple form, risk assessment divides women into high- and low-risk groups. For decades, obstetric and midwifery textbooks have published lists of potentially hazardous conditions in pregnancy with this aim; see, for example, *Principles of obstetrics* by Hibbard (1988: 172) and *Myles' textbook for midwives* (Bennett & Brown 1993: 129).

Many midwives today will be familiar with some form of risk checklist. This may take the form of a list of medical and obstetric conditions printed in the maternity notes, which both structure the booking interview, ensuring that a thorough history is taken, and alert subsequent readers of the notes to adverse conditions. Alternatively, or in addition, lists of risk factors may be published separately from the notes, as part of the maternity unit's antenatal policy. Increasingly, computers are being used to record information gathered during the booking interview, some systems highlighting any risk factors the woman may have on the print-out. Some may even generate a special list of factors present, a 'risk card' (Carroll *et al* 1988). Lists may also be divided into those factors apparent at booking and those arising during pregnancy.

In the most simple use of lists of risk factors, a woman is considered 'high risk' if she has, or develops, one or more of the factors on the list. Her subsequent care is then altered accordingly. For example, at unit A in the author's survey (Table 3.1 above), high-risk women have more antenatal check-ups than do those who are low risk, and in unit B they have consultant-led care rather than GP- or midwife-led care. In the Netherlands, there is a nationally agreed list of risk factors, the result, incidentally, of discussion between an obstetrician and the medical advisers of insurance companies (Oppenheimer 1993; Eskes & van Alten 1994) (Table 3.1 above). There, those women with none of the factors on the list ('low-risk' women) are cared for solely by their GP or a midwife and may choose either a home or a hospital birth, while the remaining 'high-risk' women are under the care of an obstetrician. Insurance companies provide reimbursement of fees for care (Oppenheimer 1993). The Dutch have used this list to divide women into risk groups since 1959.

More sophisticated than just noting the presence or absence of a risk factor on a list is risk scoring, another means of dividing women into risk categories. Numerous risk scores have been developed since the 1960s, when large computerised databases became available (Alexander & Keirse 1989). These scores give risk a numerical value: the greater the risk, the higher the score. They may be as simple as a mere count of the risk factors present, or, recognising that some factors may be more risky than others, the factors may be weighted before they are combined, so that they contribute appropriately to the overall score (Wall 1988; Chard *et al* 1990). Combination of the factors is often by addition, although it has been suggested that statistical techniques such as Bayes theorem or multiple logistic regression give better results (Chard 1991). Women are then grouped into high- and low-risk categories by assigning a cut-off point, often arbitrarily (Wall 1988).

Of the many risk scores developed, the Antenatal Prediction Score, described by Chamberlain *et al* in 1978, is one of the most simple, with the stated aim of assessing a woman's 'obstetrical potential'. It uses six risk factors, combined by addition. Many scores have more specific aims. The score of Goodwin *et al* (1969) is considered to be among the best (Wall 1988; LeFevre *et al* 1989) and aims to predict fetal death. The score of Creasy *et al* (1980) (a revised version of Papiernik's score: Papiernik-Berkhauer 1969) aims to evaluate the risk of premature labour, as does that of Ross *et al* (1986). This latter score is, however, designed to be used at the time of birth and illustrates that some scores may have more epidemiological than predictive use. Hobel's score (Hobel *et al* 1973) assesses the risk of a poor fetal outcome generally, but is complicated, involving 51 antenatal and 40 intrapartum factors. Edwards *et al* (1979) found that it took an average of 5 minutes and a five-page manual to calculate Hobel's score.

☐ **How effective is it?**

The idea of being able to divide women into high- or low-risk groups, particularly by the apparently sophisticated method of risk scoring, seems attractive. However, although several maternity units in southern England have recently developed their own list of risk factors (Table 3.1 above), none of those surveyed is using risk scores. There is little reason to suppose that these units do not reflect midwifery practice elsewhere in the country.

The very sophistication of risk scoring may be one reason why the technique of scoring is rarely used by midwives. Midwives will probably find risk assessment to be of more practical use if they gain from it guidance about the appropriateness of a referral, rather than a numerical estimate of the degree of risk. Also, despite the increasing use of computers in antenatal clinics, and even in the community, the calculation of scores is likely to be a nuisance to a busy clinician (Chard 1991).

It has also become apparent that most scores are simply not very good at predicting outcomes (Wall 1988; Alexander & Keirse 1989). No score yet seems to incorporate the ideal combination of factors and statistical techniques. The problems are compounded when, as is likely, the women for whom the score is to be used have different characteristics from those of the population from which the score was derived (Chard 1991). For example, Hobel's score was developed from a study of women in Los Angeles (Hobel *et al* 1973), who are not necessarily representative of women in other places at other times. Consequently, many scores lack *sensitivity*, meaning that they miss many pregnancies that will become complicated, and *specificity*, that is, they include in the high-risk group many women who will have normal pregnancies and labours. They also have a low *positive predictive power*; that is, the proportion of women classified as high risk who subsequently have a complicated pregnancy or labour is low (Golding & Peters 1988; Wall 1988). Thus, most women who score highly and will therefore be considered as at high risk will proceed normally through their pregnancies, while complications may well develop amongst the low scorers.

With the increasing use of lists of risk factors, it seems important to evaluate their efficiency at dividing women into risk categories. Such evaluation might be carried out by using mortality rates, a standard way to assess maternity care. However, mortality rates are a reliable assessment tool only if numbers are large (Bull 1994). Another way to assess a list's effectiveness is to consider the extent to which it achieves its, sometimes very specific, purpose. For example, if, as in the Netherlands, a list aims to separate those women who may receive all their maternity care from a GP or midwife from those needing obstetric care, the transfer rate from the former to the latter might be considered as a suitable measure of the list's efficiency.

Numerous studies of the Dutch system, which is almost unique in Europe, have been carried out over the last two decades. Amongst these, the Wormerveer study (van Alten *et al* 1989) considered 7980 women booked for midwifery care in a suburb of Amsterdam from 1969 to 1983. It found that a little over 17 per cent of these women were transferred to obstetric care during pregnancy, and a further 6.6 per cent during labour.

The Wormerveer study also considered neonatal morbidity (measured as convulsions within 48 hours of birth) and perinatal death rates, finding that rates compared favourably with those in the rest of Europe. Of the 89 perinatal deaths that occurred, only 17 per cent were of babies of women initially judged to be low risk (van Alten *et al* 1989). The Dutch do not, as yet, have a complete perinatal database, and there is evidence of under-reporting of perinatal deaths (Doornbos *et al* 1987). However, the estimated perinatal mortality rate amongst deliveries by midwives of 0.9 per 1000 total births (Oppenheimer 1993) compares very favourably with the national rate in 1991 of 9.1 per 1000 (Eskes & van Alten 1994).

Although the Dutch have been seeking to improve their list of risk criteria since 1987, particularly to allow a medium-risk category of women who, while referred to an obstetrician, will remain under the care of the midwife or GP, many consider the system in the Netherlands to be efficient (Ris 1986; Tew 1990; Kitzinger 1993; Oppenheimer 1993).

Reynolds *et al* (1988) similarly used rates of transfer to obstetric care when they questioned the continuing use of the traditional list of criteria for selection for GP care in Britain. Applying the criteria 'with some flexibility', 3386 women were identified as low risk and booked to have their babies at the GP unit within the John Radcliffe Hospital, Oxford, between 1981 and 1984. More than 20 per cent of these women were referred to the obstetric unit during their pregnancies, and a further (approximately) 12 per cent were transferred in labour.

Reynolds *et al* (1988) felt that these transfer rates were high, indicating that the selection process of women for care at the GP unit was poor. They suggested that the criteria might be improved by including social class, weight and smoking, thus reducing the number of women initially being classified as low risk. However, they felt that even this would only bring a slight reduction in these transfer rates.

More recently, a Scottish study to compare midwifery-led and consultant-led care also used low-risk criteria based on the recommendations of 1959, and also found high transfer rates to obstetric management (Hundley *et al* 1994). Of the 2844 women booking at Aberdeen Maternity Hospital between October 1991 and December 1992, 1900 were randomised to deliver in the midwives' unit. Thirty-four per cent of these were transferred antenatally, and a further 16 per cent during labour.

Again, the conclusion was drawn that these traditional criteria are unable to identify women who will remain at low risk throughout pregnancy and labour. However, Jones (1995) points out that over 60 per cent of these women proceeded to have straightforward deliveries. Although he suggests that these women were therefore transferred unnecessarily, it is possible that the transfers were, in fact, appropriate and that complications were prevented by timely intervention.

Whether transfer rates accurately reflect the efficiency of risk criteria thus remains debatable. It has also been suggested that high antenatal transfer rates indicate that the service allows choices to be made (Macfarlane 1994), an issue that will be discussed later.

It is difficult to draw conclusions about the efficiency of methods to divide women into risk groups; the feeling of the Royal College of Obstetricians and Gynaecologists in 1992 was that no method was, as things then stood, sufficiently reliable. However, many recently introduced schemes of maternity care are currently being evaluated, often including an assessment of the risk criteria used. Results will be awaited with interest.

□ **Why is it not more effective?**

Risk assessment is obviously at its best when based on maximum information. Thus it will be more accurate the later it is done in pregnancy (Rosen *et al* 1978). Similarly, prediction of complications is better for multiparous than for primigravid women, simply because the most reliable risk factors are those relating to previous obstetric history, of which primigravidae have none (Bull 1994; Cole & McIlwaine 1994). Illustrating this, only 4 per cent of primigravid women in a recent Scottish study were judged to be at high risk at booking, compared with 26 per cent of multiparous women. However, of the remaining low-risk women, almost twice as many primigravidae as multiparae developed complications requiring delivery in hospital (Cole & McIlwaine 1994).

Incorrect use of a risk assessment scheme that is unfamiliar may also cause women to be wrongly allocated to risk groups. Both Breyer and Stolk (1971) and Smits (1975) felt that the Dutch list of risk factors was being used inappropriately in its early years.

Furthermore, even when midwives do identify risk factors in their booking interviews, studies in Scotland, Leeds and London have shown that the information may be subsequently ignored or not appropriately acted upon by other health care professionals (Chng *et al* 1980; Guthrie *et al* 1989; Yoong *et al* 1992).

Finally, many complications of pregnancy may simply prove never to be predictable (Chng *et al* 1980).

☐ **How helpful is it?**

There are doubts about how accurately women with high-risk pregnancies can be identified. There are also questions about whether it really is helpful to identify them and whether the 'intrusion into the privacy of the pregnant woman' (Alexander & Keirse 1989), required by many of the methods of assessing risk, is really warranted. Whether women are rightly or wrongly identified – effectively, 'labelled' – the effects on them fall into three categories.

First, a 'label' of high risk, which may be as literal as some mark, such as a star or red cross on the pregnancy notes (many of which are now held by expectant mothers; Magill-Cuerden 1992), may have psychological or emotional effects on the woman. She may feel that she is different from other women and feel odd, embarrassed, anxious or distressed (Aikins Murphy 1994). She may feel inadequate or worried that she is failing her unborn child in some way, and guilty if she persists in 'risky' behaviour, such as smoking, or even over circumstances that are outside her control, such as poor housing. The stress caused by assigning her to a high-risk group may itself provoke complications (Alexander & Keirse 1989; Oakley 1992).

Being considered 'high risk' also almost inevitably leads to extra interventions, such as advice, investigation or treatment. The benefits of many such interventions, even for correctly 'labelled' women, are now being questioned (Aikins Murphy 1994). For most pregnancies, sophisticated technology is totally inappropriate and can cause feelings of loss of control, and sometimes considerable emotional and physical discomfort (Styles 1994). With many women being labelled as 'high risk' in error, large numbers of normal expectant mothers are having their experience of pregnancy and childbirth thus compromised.

Finally, not only might a high-risk woman receive too much attention because of her risk status, but she may also miss some of the benefits of low-risk care, particularly the continuity that a midwife or GP can provide.

These negative effects could be minimised for some 'high-risk' women if, once it is clear that their threatened complications will not arise or have been resolved, they were returned to the low-risk group. Unfortunately, this often does not happen (Hall 1990).

■ Dealing with antenatal risks today

There appear to be two major changes with implications for risk assessment taking place in maternity care today, at least in the UK.

First, as maternity units seek to implement the recommendations of *Changing childbirth* (DoH 1993), systems of care are likely to change so that each woman will have a lead professional responsible for her care. This professional may be a midwife, GP or obstetrician, depending on the mother's preference and on whether or not medical or obstetric problems are apparent at her booking appointment. Such a professional will provide the mother with continuity, while also ensuring that referrals are made to, and care given by, others as appropriate. The CRAG/SCOTMEG Working Group on Maternity Services in Scotland considers that 'all women are suitable for midwife or general practitioner antenatal care' (Scottish Office 1995: 15), with obstetricians becoming involved in the care of women who have a risk factor requiring specialist attention. Such new systems of care will avoid categorising women into high- and low-risk groups and will thus also avoid 'labelling' women as in some way different or abnormal.

Second, computers are becoming commonplace rather than exceptional in antenatal clinics and are also being used by some midwives in the community (Maresh 1990). Doubts have been expressed about the quality of the relationship developed between the mother and the midwife when a computer is used at the interview (Methven 1990). Indeed, Brownbridge *et al* (1988) have shown that when computers are used at booking interviews, midwives tend to spend longer taking histories, ask more closed questions, and spend more time attending to records and less exclusively to the expectant mother, giving less advice. However, they also found that the length of time for which midwives give women their undivided attention increased with experience in the use of the computer, women generally feeling that the computer did not affect the interview, and midwives being keen to continue using the technology.

Computers are certainly able to record more information, with more detail, than is possible with most manual systems (Lilford *et al* 1990). By prompting appropriate questions, they can also structure the history taking process so that no relevant information is missed or irrelevancies asked. Thus, computers can assist accurate and thorough record keeping and, as long as the information held on them is easily accessible, usually on a printout, they can also aid good communication amongst those involved in the expectant mother's care. A computerised system of action suggestions has been proposed (Lilford & Chard 1983) and is currently being developed by Fawdry (pers comm 1995), in which, in response to the details entered, the computer produces a list of suggested investigations or treatments and optimum times for carrying them out. Whether the provision of such action suggestions really will lead to improved standards of antenatal care, as seems to be the case in general medicine (McDonald 1976), has yet to be shown (Lilford *et al* 1990).

The most important features of risk assessment now appear to be the identification of problems, the recording of information and the relaying of that information to all concerned, so that the problems are dealt with in the most appropriate manner. Thus, good risk assessment is analogous with good antenatal care. It is not necessary to discuss the importance of the midwife being thorough and skilful in her history taking and subsequent antenatal examinations, accurate and complete in her record keeping, whether assisted by computer or not, up to date and relevant in her knowledge, sensitive to, and understanding of, the expectant mother, unbiased and informative in her explanations, and professional and co-operative when considering subsequent care. However, two questions seem to persist in the minds of those caring for women antenatally, as considered below.

☐ **What constitutes a significant risk?**

As mentioned before, this is an age-old question, the answer to which will probably never be agreed to everyone's satisfaction.

Most clinicians would, however, agree that certain broad categories of risk factor must be considered in any assessment of risk. The likelihood of problems arising is known to vary with parity, age, physique, family history, smoking habits and socioeconomic circumstances (Hall 1990), and such factors would therefore be likely to be included in some way. Any medical disorder can affect, or be affected by, a pregnancy and should therefore be noted as requiring regular and careful assessment (US Department of Health and Human Services 1989). Previous obstetric history should also be taken into account, as some pregnancy problems may recur or adversely affect subsequent pregnancies (Hall 1990). Obviously, problems in the current pregnancy need to be dealt with as they arise.

Although most of the risk factors customarily considered by midwives are given in Table 3.1 above, the relative contribution of each to risk remains largely subjective. Some studies have been carried out to try to ascertain this more objectively, but, as appropriate control groups are needed and very large data sets are usually required, such studies are hard to conduct (Hall 1990; Chard 1991).

Having up to date knowledge is vital as risk factors can, and do, change (Oakley 1992; Mendez-Bauer *et al* 1994). The negative effects of many risk factors, such as Rhesus isoimmunisation and unmarried motherhood, for example, are decreasing. Furthermore, other risks, such as the increases in the use of social drugs and in the incidence of AIDS, are acquiring more significance. Perhaps forensic risk, where obstetrics is practised defensively to avoid litigation rather than in the best interests of the expectant mother and her unborn baby, should also be included amongst these. The increasing rates of caesarean section in some Western countries, for example from 10.5 per cent in England and Wales in 1985 (Francome *et al* 1993) to a probable rate of 15.3 per cent in 1993 (Francome *et al* 1994), may be evidence that forensic risk is increasingly real.

The best way to deal with this question of what constitutes a significant risk is to keep abreast of current research into enumeration of the risks in pregnancy and to draw on the experience of others.

☐ **Risk and choice – are these mutually exclusive?**

In the UK, the Expert Maternity Group identified the first principle of good maternity care as 'The woman must be the focus of maternity care. She should be able to feel that she is in control of what is happening to her and able to make decisions about her care' (DoH 1993: 8).

The idea of giving women choice in their maternity care has, however, prompted much discussion, some feeling that to do so might increase risks (see, for example, Chapter 11 in Chamberlain and Patel 1994: 89–99). Debate has centred on whether women really want choice or merely involvement, whether they are able to comprehend the issues involved and to articulate their desires accurately, and whether they really want, and are capable of carrying, the responsibility that accompanies choice.

However, the point has already been made that risk is very subjective (Handwerker 1994). Values, hopes and expectations are also very personal. It seems a reasonable assumption that all involved in a woman's maternity care, including the expectant mother herself, would wish for a happy and healthy outcome to her pregnancy. In cases in which a woman's choice appears to conflict with the advice of her caregivers, it seems more likely that she has weighed up the risks and benefits differently from them, rather than that she has a conflict of interests.

■ **Recommendations for clinical practice in the light of currently available evidence**

Despite the current paucity of valid and practical conclusions that can be drawn from research into risk assessment, some practical points arise from considering current trends in maternity care. These are largely covered in the text and summarized below.

1. *Individual assessment* – Risks for each pregnant woman need to be assessed individually. Understanding each woman depends, on the one hand, on forming a relationship with her and, on the other, on the sensitive gathering of relevant information from her.

2. *The booking interview* – The importance of the booking interview for both of these functions must not be underestimated. Ideally, the midwife involved should be the one who continues the woman's maternity care.

3. *Lists of risk factors*

   ● Compilation of, and use of, a list of risk factors, while never exhaustive, can give risk assessment a more objective dimension. This list must always be available to all involved in the woman's care.

   ● A list must, however, also allow for clinical judgement. Thus, good antenatal risk assessment requires relevant and up to date knowledge, sound clinical skills and the ability to anticipate problems, and must be maintained from the first contact with the pregnant woman until after delivery.

   ● The purpose of any list of risk factors needs to be clearly defined as this will dictate, to some extent, the factors to be included. For example, Table 3.1 above shows that maternity unit G has produced two lists for midwives to use, with very different purposes and different risk factors included.

   ● A list should also be locally agreed, as its content will depend partly on local facilities and circumstances (Scottish Office 1995). For example, units B and C in Table 3.1 are consultant units with specialist medical services, where factors such as high parity, short stature and being overweight are considered less of a problem than they might be elsewhere. Unit E, however, includes as risky more factors arising in pregnancy or labour than most, perhaps because it is a midwifery unit that is geographically distanced from medical care.

   ● A list of risk factors should also be based on research findings and other lists that appear to work. The suggestion of 'generally accepted criteria, applied locally' (Oppenheimer 1993: 1401) could be considered concurrently with the development of a national pregnancy health record.

4. *Professional co-operation* – By whatever means risk is assessed or problems identified, there needs to be respect and co-operation between the medical, midwifery and other professions, and clear referral systems. Referral systems need to have the flexibility to allow

the most suitably skilled professional, who is not necessarily the obstetrician (Hall 1990), to be involved.

5. *Record keeping* – Thorough record keeping is vital and can be simplified by using a list or a computer. It is important also to record the risks discussed with the expectant mother, as well as any other risk factors considered but not listed.

6. *Women's choice*

   • For women to be able to make choices in their maternity care, midwives must have the skills and knowledge to be able to communicate accurate and unbiased information to them.

   • Occasionally, a midwife may feel that, despite clear information being given, by others as well as by herself, a woman is making inappropriately risky choices. 'If this situation arises you must . . . consult as soon as possible with your supervisor of midwives, making a detailed record of the circumstances and action taken' (UKCC 1994: 9).

7. *Changing concept of risk* – Systems of care that depend on women being considered as high or low risk should be discontinued in favour of those dependent on women's choices, particularly of their lead professional (Scottish Office 1995).

■ Practice check

• Do you see the booking interview primarily as an information gathering exercise or as the basis on which you will form an ongoing relationship with an expectant mother? Does this affect how you conduct the interview?

• Do you ever find yourself writing phrases such as 'no significant problems' rather than documenting fully the risk factors you have considered?

• Do you keep your knowledge up to date and research based by reading professional journals and using the Cochrane Collaboration Pregnancy and Childbirth Database?

• If your unit has a list of risk factors, do you always use it? Do you also consider possible risks that are not included?

• What would you include on a list of risk factors? Why? What would be the purpose of your list?

• Consider how you might explain, for example, the benefits and hazards of a home birth to a woman with a history of retained placenta who is expecting her second baby.

☐ Acknowledgements

Thanks are due to many but particularly to the midwives of the maternity units who contributed details of their systems of risk assessment, and to my husband, Bill, for his encouragement and assistance.

■ References

Alexander S, Keirse MJNC 1989 Formal risk scoring during pregnancy. In Chalmers I, Enkin M, Keirse MJNC (eds) Effective care in pregnancy and childbirth. Oxford University Press, Oxford, Ch 22, p345–65

American College of Obstetricians and Gynecologists 1992 Professional liability survey highlights claims experience, merits, duration. ACOG Newsletter 36: 1–4

Andolsek KM 1993 Obstetric risk assessment. Primary Care 20(3): 551–84

Backett EM, Davies AM, Petros-Barvazian A 1984 The risk approach in health care. With special reference to maternal and child health, including family planning. Public Health Papers No. 76. World Health Organization, Geneva

Bennett VR, Brown LK (eds) 1993 Myles' textbook for midwives, 12th edn. Churchill Livingstone, London

Breyer HBG, Stolk JG 1971 Enkele beschouwingen naar aanleiding van een onderzoek over doodgeboorte in her jaar 1961 in Nederland. Ned Tijdschr Geneeskd 115: 1638–46 (English abstract)

Brownbridge G, Lilford RJ, Tindale-Biscoe S 1988 Use of a computer to take booking histories in a hospital antenatal clinic. Medical Care 26 (5): 474–87

Bull MJV 1994 Selection of women for community obstetric care. In Chamberlain G, Patel N (eds) The future of the maternity services. RCOG Press, London, Ch 9, p73–81

Carroll S, Chard T, Lloyd DS, Bradshaw J, Hudson CN, Sloan D, Griffiths S 1988 Preparation of risk cards using a computerised obstetric information system. Journal of Obstetrics and Gynaecology 8(3): 222–7

Chamberlain G, Patel N (eds) 1994 The future of the maternity services. RCOG Press, London

Chamberlain G, Philipp E, Howlett B, Masters K (1978) British births 1970. A survey under the joint auspices of the National Birthday Trust Fund and the Royal College of Obstetricians and Gynaecologists, Vol 2: Obstetric care. William Heinemann, London

Chard T (1991) Obstetric risk scores. Fetal Medicine Review 3: 1–10

Chard T, Harding S, Carroll S, Hudson CN, Lloyd DSL, Sloan D 1990 A comparison of different methods for calculating overall risk scores from risk factors ascertained in a computerized obstetric information system. Journal of Perinatal Medicine 18(1): 23–9

Chard T, Yoong A, Macintosh M (1994) Antepartum risk scores. In van Geijn HP, Copray FJA (eds) A critical appraisal of fetal surveillance. Excerpta Medica, Amsterdam, Ch 5, p34–46

Chng PK, Hall MH, MacGillivray I 1980 An audit of antenatal care: the value of the first antenatal visit. British Medical Journal 281(6249): 1184–6

Cole SK, McIlwaine GM 1994 The use of risk factors in predicting possible consequences of changing patterns of care in pregnancy. In Chamberlain G, Patel N (eds) The future of the maternity services. RCOG Press, London, Ch 8, p65–72

Creasy RK, Gummer BA, Liggins GC 1980 System for predicting spontaneous preterm birth. Obstetrics and Gynecology 55: 692–5

Department of Health 1993 Changing childbirth. Report of the Expert Maternity Group. HMSO, London

Dimond B 1994 Water births – the legal implications for midwives. Modern Midwife 4(1): 12–13

Donnai D 1988 Genetic risk. In James DK, Stirrat GM (eds) Pregnancy and risk. The basis for rational management. John Wiley, Chichester, Ch 3, p23–43

Doornbos JPR, Hendrik JN, Treffers PE 1987 The reliability of perinatal mortality statistics in The Netherlands. American Journal of Obstetrics and Gynecology 156: 1183–7

Downe S 1994 How average is normality? British Journal of Midwifery 2(7): 303–4

Edwards L E, Barrada I, Tatreau RW, Hakanson EY 1979 A simplified antepartum risk-scoring system. Obstetrics and Gynecology 54(2): 237–40

Enkin MW 1994 Risk in pregnancy: the reality, the perception, and the concept. Birth 21(3): 131–4

Eskes M, van Alten D (1994) Review and assessment of maternity services in the Netherlands. In Chamberlain G, Patel N (eds) The future of the maternity services. RCOG Press, London, Ch 4, p36–46

Francome C, Savage W, Churchill H, Lewison H 1993 Caesarean birth in Britain: a book for health professionals and parents. Middlesex University Press, London

Francome C, Savage W, Lewison H 1994 Caesarean birth in Britain (1994 supplement). National Childbirth Trust and Middlesex University Press, London

Golding J, Peters TJ 1988 Quantifying risk in pregnancy. In James DK, Stirrat GM (eds) pregnancy and risk. The basis for rational management. John Wiley, Chichester, Ch 2, p7–22

Goodwin JW, Dunne JT, Thomas BW 1969 Antepartum identification of the fetus at risk. Canadian Medical Association Journal 101(8): 57–67

Guthrie KA, Songane FF, Mackenzie F, Lilford RJ 1989 Audit of medical response to antenatal booking history. British Journal of Obstetrics and Gynaecology 96(5): 552–6

Hall MH 1990 Identification of high risk and low risk. Baillière's Clinical Obstetrics and Gynaecology 4(1): 65–76

Handwerker L 1994 Medical risk: implicating poor pregnant women. Social Science and Medicine 38(5): 665–75

Hibbard BM 1988 Principles of obstetrics. Butterworth, London

Hobel CJ, Hyvarinen MA, Okada DM, Oh W 1973 Prenatal and intrapartum high risk screening. I. Prediction of the high risk neonate. American Journal of Obstetrics and Gynecology 117(1): 1–9

Hundley VA, Cruikshank FM, Lang GD, Glazener CMA, Milne JM, Turner M, Blyth D, Mollison J, Donaldson C 1994 Midwife managed delivery unit: a randomised controlled comparison with consultant led care. British Medical Journal 309(6966): 1400–4

James DK, Stirrat GM 1988 Introduction: the concept of risk. In James DK, Stirrat GM (eds) Pregnancy and risk. The basis for rational management. John Wiley, Chichester, Ch 1, p1–5

Jones IG 1995 Study shows interventionist nature of British obstetrics. British Medical Journal 310(6982): 806 (letter)

Kitzinger S 1993 Change in midwifery – a cross-cultural view. Modern Midwife 3(3): 4–5

LeFevre M, Williamson HA, Hector M Jr 1989 Obstetric risk assessment in rural practice. Journal of Family Practice 28(6): 691–6

Lilford RJ, Chard T 1983 Problems and pitfalls of risk assessment in antenatal care. British Journal of Obstetrics and Gynaecology 906(6): 507–10

Lilford RJ, Guthrie K, Kelly M 1990 History-taking by computer. Baillière's Clinical Obstetrics and Gynaecology 4(4): 723–42

Lilford RJ, Kelly M, Baines A, Cameron S, Cave M, Guthrie K, Thornton J 1992 Effects of using protocols on medical care: randomised trial of three methods of taking an antenatal history. British Medical Journal 305(6863): 1181–4

Lloyd GER (ed.) 1983 Hippocratic writings. Penguin Classics, Harmondsworth

McDonald CJ 1976 Protocol-based computer reminders, the quality of care and the non-perfectability of man. New England Journal of Medicine 295(24): 1351–4

Macfarlane A 1994 Comment made in: Balancing risks and choice: Discussion. In Chamberlain G, Patel N (eds) The future of the maternity services. RCOG Press, London, Ch 11, p89–99

Magill-Cuerden J 1992 A question of communication. Modern Midwife 2(6): 4–5

Maresh M 1990 The use of computers in the provision of care during childbirth. Midwifery 6(1): 41–8

Mendez-Bauer C, Almagro Martinez J, Segura M, Luna J, Mendez-Bauer F, Zamarriego J 1994 The profile of perinatal risk factors. In van Geijn HP, Copray FJA (eds) A critical appraisal of fetal surveillance. Excerpta Medica, Amsterdam, Ch 19, p151–7

Methven RC 1990 The antenatal booking interview. In Alexander J, Levy V, Roch S (eds) Antenatal care: a research based approach. Macmillan, Basingstoke, Ch 3, p42–57

Ministry of Health 1959 Report of the Maternity Services Committee (the Cranbrook Committee report). HMSO, London

Moore PG 1983 The business of risk. Cambridge University Press, Cambridge

Murphy P Aikins 1994 Risk, risk assessment and risk labels. Journal of Nurse–Midwifery 39(2): 67–9

Oakley A 1992 Social support and motherhood. The natural history of a research project. Blackwell, Oxford

Office of Population Censuses and Surveys 1994 OPCS Monitor, 21 December: 4

Oppenheimer C 1993 Organising midwifery led care in the Netherlands. British Medical Journal 307(6916): 1400–2

Page LA 1994 Opening remarks to: Balancing risks and choice: Discussion. In Chamberlain G, Patel N (eds) The future of the maternity services. RCOG Press, London, Ch 11, p89–99

Papiernik-Berkhauer E 1969 Coefficient de risque d'accouchement prématuré (C.R.A.P.). Presse Medicale 77(21): 793–4

Reynolds JL, Yudkin PL, Bull MJV 1988 General practitioner obstetrics: does risk prediction work? Journal of the Royal College of General Practitioners 38(312): 307–10

Ris M 1986 Obstetrical care in The Netherlands. The place of midwives and specific aspects of their rôle. In Kuminski M, Bréart G, Buekens P, Huisjes HJ, McIlwaine G, Selbmann H (eds) Perinatal care delivery systems. Oxford University Press, Oxford, Ch 11, p167–77

Rosen MG, Sokol RJ, Chik L 1978 Use of computers in the labor and delivery suite: an overview. American Journal of Obstetrics and Gynecology 132(6): 589–94

Ross MG, Hobel CJ, Bragonier JR, Bear MB, Bemis RL 1986 A simplified risk-scoring system for prematurity. American Journal of Perinatology 3(4): 339–44

Royal College of Obstetricians and Gynaecologists 1992 Complete response of the Royal College of Obstetricians and Gynaecologists to the Report of the House of Commons Health Committee on Maternity Services. RCOG, London

Scherger JE 1988 Commentary. Journal of Family Practice 27(2): 162–3

Scottish Office 1995 Antenatal care. Report of the CRAG/SCOTMEG Working Group on Maternity Services, Edinburgh: HMSO

Scottish Office Home and Health Department 1993 Provision of maternity services in Scotland. A policy review. HMSO, Edinburgh

Smits F 1975 The efficacy of the selection process of obstetrical care. PhD thesis, University of Nijmegen, Holland (in Dutch, with French abstract)

Steer PJ 1994 Risks and complications. Paper given at The Future of the Maternity Services meeting, 14 October 1994, organised jointly by the RCOG, RCM and RCGP at the Royal College of Obstetricians and Gynaecologists

Styles WMcN 1994 Opening remarks to: Balancing technology with non-intervention: Discussion. In Chamberlain G, Patel N (eds) The future of the maternity services. RCOG Press, London, Ch 22, p166–75

Tew M 1990 Safer childbirth? A critical history of maternity care. Chapman & Hall, London

United Kingdom Central Council for Nursing, Midwifery and Health Visiting 1993 Midwives' rules. UKCC, London

United Kingdom Central Council for Nursing, Midwifery and Health Visiting 1994 The midwife's code of practice. UKCC, London

US Department of Health and Human Services 1989 Caring for our future: the content of prenatal care. A Report of the Public Health Service Expert Panel on the content of prenatal care. US Department of Health and Human Services, Washington, DC

van Alten D, Eskes M, Treffers PE 1989 Midwifery in the Netherlands. The Wormerveer study: selection, model of delivery, perinatal mortality and infant morbidity. British Journal of Obstetrics and Gynaecology 96(6): 656–62

Wall EM 1988 Assessing obstetric risk. A review of obstetric risk-scoring systems. Journal of Family Practice 27(2): 153–63

Whelton J 1993 Fetal medicine. In Alexander J, Levy V, Roch S (eds) Midwifery practice: a research-based approach. Macmillan, Basingstoke, Ch 4, p55–73

Yoong AFE, Lim J, Hudson CN, Chard T 1992 Audit of compliance with antenatal protocols. British Medical Journal   305(6863): 1184–6

■ Suggested further reading

Alexander S, Keirse MJNC 1989 Formal risk scoring during pregnancy. In Chalmers I, Enkin M, Keirse MJNC (eds) Effective care in pregnancy and childbirth. Oxford University Press, Oxford, Ch 22, p345–65

Chamberlain G, Patel N (eds) 1994 The future of the maternity services. RCOG Press, London

James DK, Stirrat GM (eds) 1988 Pregnancy and risk. The basis for rational management. John Wiley, Chichester

Oakley A 1992 Social support and motherhood. The natural history of a research project. Blackwell, Oxford, Ch 10

Oakley A, Houd S 1990 Helpers in childbirth: midwifery today. Hemisphere Publishing Corporation, New York, Ch 6 (p115–31) and 7 (p133 –60)

Chapter 4

Antenatal education, health promotion and the midwife

Colin Rees

Antenatal education has frequently been seen as a challenge for midwifery (Murphy-Black 1990). Now, with the increased emphasis on health promotion (DoH 1992), the complexity of working with women has increased even further. Uncertainty exists in the minds of midwives and managers over the continued allocation of scarce midwifery resources to these activities, especially antenatal classes. Do they benefit women, their babies and the service? If they do, how can we demonstrate this?

This chapter examines some of the evidence relating to antenatal education since the work of Murphy-Black (1990) and attempts to answer the questions 'Is antenatal education moving forwards?' and 'Can its value be clearly demonstrated?' The discussion will then be broadened to consider the issue of health promotion in an attempt to clarify the implications for the midwife.

The literature is mainly based on British sources. An attempt has been made to avoid repetition of the previous work of Murphy-Black (1990) by limiting the review to work published after the late 1980s. Inevitably, some of the classic publications in the field will still be mentioned.

It will be seen that the subject continues to be under-researched and that work that does exist is often open to methodological criticism. Nevertheless, there is a feeling of optimism regarding midwifery potential surrounding its role in antenatal classes and health promotion. This potential will only be achieved, however, if the weaknesses of the past are taken into account, and providing that the new directions reported here continue to be supported by health service managers.

■ **It is assumed that you are already aware of the following:**

- The basic principles of adult education;
- Techniques of group work;

58

- Antenatal education skills;

- Participatory learning principles;

- Approaches to health promotion;

- Interpersonal communication skills.

◼ Antenatal education - are we moving forwards?

In the late 1970s and early 1980s, there was a great deal of published work on antenatal education, particularly covering consumer views on antenatal classes. A number of issues were examined, including the characteristics of those who attended, the nature of the classes and the approaches and skills of those responsible for providing them (Perkins 1980).

It was acknowledged that classes suffered from a number of problems, including a low attendance rate, a high drop-out rate, a selective group attending and dissatisfaction amongst both midwives and health visitors with their involvement in them (Rees 1982). In Murphy-Black's (1990) review of the literature that covers this period, the following factors were given as reasons for poor attendance at antenatal classes:

- Clients did not want to go;

- Clients did not know about them;

- Clients thought classes not worthwhile;

- Clients thought exercise might harm the baby;

- Clients felt confident without attending;

- Too costly;

- Poor timing in the day;

- Poor transport or location difficult;

- Clients attended in previous pregnancy;

- No provision for children.

Has midwifery addressed some of these issues in the intervening years? It has to be said that, apart from some published new initiatives on a local level (Clements 1989; Dunwoody & Watters 1990; Turner 1993), very little seems to have happened as far as the literature is concerned. Following the flood of interest around the turn of the 1980s and the seminal work of people such as Perkins (1978, 1979, 1980), there has been a slowing down of the research interest in the subject. This led Rees

(1993) to ask whether midwifery had lost interest in antenatal classes. He demonstrated, using a small group of 15 midwives, that the problems of poor attendance and the challenge of producing lively sessions at antenatal classes still existed.

☐ **The relevance of antenatal classes**

In this section, the issue of the benefits of antenatal classes will be examined. However, we must first consider the purpose of classes and question whether they are still relevant in the present midwifery service.

It should be noted that there has been no report in the literature of any decline in the provision of antenatal classes. It still seems likely, then, that we can use the words of Simkin and Enkin (1989) to say that they represent a significant and widespread intervention in pregnancy care today. In this, the midwife plays a substantial role (O'Connor 1993), although we must acknowledge the continually well-evaluated role of other participants such as the National Childbirth Trust (Davies 1989).

Are classes any different now from what they used to be? According to Simkin and Enkin (1989), antenatal education has become more complex as it has expanded beyond its primary goal of two and three decades ago of reducing pain in labour. However, they observe that the aims can differ widely from class to class and from teacher to teacher, depending on the philosophy of those involved.

A number of aims have been claimed for classes. Some provide what might be termed the traditional function of preparation for birth. Even where initiatives have been launched to improve classes, professionals still see this as their major role. This was demonstrated in a small study by Clements (1989), who set up a multidisciplinary working group to assess the problems, concerns and needs of present-day mothers. Unfortunately, no mothers were involved in the study. The work of the group revolved around a review of the literature and a survey of local midwives and health visitors to determine issues that they felt required further exploration. Although a number of relevant issues were identified, the group recommended that the theme of the classes should remain preparation for labour. It was agreed, however, that the classes should be structured more towards the needs and expectations of the mothers attending the classes.

Other writers have seen the scope for classes as being wider than simply preparation for labour. O'Connor (1993), for instance, comments that preparation for parenthood classes in both hospitals and the community provide an ideal opportunity for prospective parents to learn about the many aspects of parenthood. The social function of classes in bringing people in a similar situation together and taking advantage of what they can learn from each other has also been identified as a further possibility. So, for instance, Rees (1993: 75) makes the following point:

> One feasible aim is to provide an opportunity for those in a similar situation to come together, to obtain answers to questions and uncertainties in a supportive atmosphere, and to learn from the concerns of others. It is also possible to sensitise those who attend to some of the issues and options relating to pregnancy and child care. In this way, classes can empower women as far as possible within the limits of their own personal circumstances and the limitations of the health service.

For most people, classes are places where information is provided and where certain skills, such as breathing and relaxation to reduce pain in labour, are learnt. Simkin and Enkin (1989) also suggest their potential role as 'a vehicle for attitude modification, towards on the one hand increased self-reliance and questioning on the part of the woman or couple, or on the other to increased compliance with and adherence to prescribed medical regimens'. Although this implies the possible use of classes as a way of gaining conformity to a professional-led system of care, they do go on to say 'all classes have as their goal to enhance each woman's sense of optimism and confidence as she approaches childbirth'.

From this examination of the aims of classes, we can characterise their purpose as one of 'preparation', which is how most people unquestioningly think of them. There are two aspects of this: first, physical preparation, and, second, what Cogan (1983) referred to as 'diffuse mental hygiene'. Under this heading, Cogan includes such items as anxiety reduction, positive attitudes toward pregnancy, knowledge, labour support and emotional satisfaction.

☐ **Problem areas**

Following all that has been written on the potential of antenatal education and the recommendations for its improvement, it is disappointing to find O'Connor (1993: 199) pondering:

> Why is that for over 11 years the same conclusions have been drawn from within the profession and from outside, yet change only occurs in isolated areas leaving the majority of expectant parents with second-rate, inflexible, out-dated classes?

One of the main problems suggested by O'Connor is the content of classes. She suggests that there is still a search for a format that is interesting and useful, as assessed by prospective parents. Looking at the literature, she concludes that the overwhelming view that emerges is the need to tailor the content of the classes to the needs of the consumer.

Combes and Schonveld (1992), in their comprehensive critical review of the relevant literature, also identify a number of problem areas that have been raised in various studies. These are (page 31):

- Lack of teaching about childcare;
- Poor coverage of understanding about parenting;
- Failure to dispel unrealistic expectations;
- Lack of advice on how to avoid negative feelings and experiences;
- Unrealistic preparation for labour;
- Failure to recognise the differing circumstances of individuals.

Many of these problems seem to be related to the philosophical approach of the midwives and their understanding of the purpose of classes. Rees (1993) points out that one of the difficulties is that the historical tradition of providing classes means that they have become taken for granted. Rarely, says Rees, do midwives stop to ask the question 'What are they for?' He goes on to suggest that without being clear on the rationale behind them, the midwife is frequently left to follow a well-worn routine of 'talk' and 'exercises'.

This issue has been pursued by a number of commentators who have tried to answer the question 'Whose agenda do classes follow?' Combes and Schonveld's (1992) research, based on interviews with 18 health professionals in group discussions, found that a strong and recurring theme was that health professionals wanted to work to the agenda of pregnant women.

However, they found that there was an ambivalence concerning how far the agendas of women should influence the content of classes. An entirely women-led agenda was seen by most of the respondents as not desirable. The view expressed was that pregnant women do not always know their own needs, and that part of the health professional's role is to present what, from past experience, women ought to find useful. The respondents also felt that they had a legitimate professional agenda, based on the priorities of the health service, to which they needed to work and for which they were accountable.

There are two main problems with this study. First, is it based on small numbers, and second, there is no indication that those in the sample are representative of those involved in parent education.

Nevertheless, the theme of 'whose agenda' is also found in the literature from other countries such as New Zealand (Gilkison 1991). Through a clear analysis of the problems in her own country, Gilkison identifies a number of issues that sound very familiar. She begins by stating that the broad aim of antenatal education in New Zealand is to allow pregnant women and their partners to learn about fetal development and maternal health during pregnancy, to prepare for childbirth and to teach parenting skills.

The classes, she says, are often large and are usually held in maternity units for those in late pregnancy. Classes may be taught by midwives, childbirth educators or physiotherapists. They are normally held in the hospital environment and prepare couples for the kind of birth they can expect in a New Zealand hospital. Gilkison points out that the institution that offers the classes has a high level of control over them, deciding for whom the classes will be provided, what should be taught, who should teach it and how they will be evaluated.

The answer to the question 'Whose agenda is being addressed?' is made clear in the choice of words Gilkison uses to describe the nature of the sessions, as the following passage illustrates:

> Much of the material covered in classes aims to 'prepare' women for childbirth in that particular institution. In other words, admission procedures will be 'described', technological devices and possible interventions will be 'explained', women will be told what to 'expect' from various staff members, how they will feel at certain stages of labour and what will be *done* to help them. Women are encouraged to ask questions about the procedures, and offered 'choices' within certain boundaries, but to question the status quo or to challenge the system is definitely not a part of most antenatal classes. Preparation for childbirth then, could be analogous with shaping a woman's behaviour to accommodate the requirements of the institution.
>
> (Gilkison 1991: 13)

It is clear from this that women are expected to be passive and that the aim of the sessions is very much that of social control: to get women to fit into the system. The way in which the information is presented, in terms of whether it is offered as a topic for debate or whether there are no options available, will influence how women respond to the sessions. It will also influence how they perceive their own role and the extent to which they feel that this is defined for them in pregnancy and labour generally.

This is a point that has been made by Simkin and Enkin (1989: 320), who observe that:

> Depending on the ideology, preferences, and biases of the teacher, antenatal education may either promote or discourage parent decision making, use of medications, acceptance of routine interventions or alternatives, formula or breast feeding, and anxiety or confidence in the caregiver and place of birth.

This does not, perhaps, do women justice in the way it regards them as lacking the ability to reject the views of the professional. Nevertheless, it does highlight the importance of the beliefs of the midwife regarding her role, particularly if that includes the view that what she puts forward is the 'right' view and should not be challenged.

☐ **Introducing change**

One of the first important stages in improving antenatal classes is to recognise that there is a need to change them. In their research, Combes and Schonveld (1992) found that professionals involved with parent education felt that there was a general resistance by those involved in the system to change. This was seen as an obstacle to thinking about how well classes meet women's needs. Those in the study felt there was an attitude held by others that 'We've always done it this way and no one's ever complained', or that women turning up to classes was proof that everything was all right as it was.

The study also found that several respondents felt there was a tendency to add topics to classes, not on the basis of need but because there was someone locally who could come and 'do a good session' on a particular topic. In this situation, those attending are simply seen as a passive 'audience' who should be 'talked at'.

Here the problem is that of the didactic style sometimes adopted by teachers (Hillan 1994). Under these conditions, it is highly unlikely that the individual attending will have her needs satisfied. This is particularly problematic where there is a variety of different needs within the group. Hillan goes on to make the following observation:

> Inevitably antenatal classes will have participants of mixed needs and abilities and good antenatal teaching requires staff to be responsive to the needs of individual women and their partners. This involves allowing the participants to direct the choice of topics to be discussed – taking a proactive rather than reactive approach.
>
> (Hillan 1994: 62)

The major theme of much of the literature on improving antenatal classes, particularly those on running classes, is the participatory style required in sessions if needs are to be identified (Murphy-Black & Faulkner 1988; Priest & Schott 1991).

It is easy to suggest changes such as this, but there is the problem of whether midwives necessarily have the skills to implement them. Murphy-Black (1990), for instance, makes the point that although much of midwifery involves teaching, the main skills are frequently those of one-to-one teaching, whereas teaching a group demands different skills.

Is there evidence from the literature to suggest that changes can be successfully introduced? Although a number of changes may have been introduced into antenatal classes in recent years, very few have been submitted for publication so that others may learn from the initiatives. There are, however, three exceptions (Clements 1989; Dunwoody & Watters 1990; Turner 1993). These three examples have a number of common elements. They were each embarked upon as a result of a dissatisfaction with the current way of conducting sessions. They all established a working group to design the form of the innovation. There was also a common move away from didactic teaching to participatory learning methods, with the midwife acting as facilitator.

It is also worth commenting on the enthusiasm of each of the writers for the innovations and the fact that the new approach was found to be favourably received by women attending sessions. All of them, however, have the weakness that they are poorly evaluated. This is an important area, as we shall see from the next section.

☐ Evaluation of antenatal classes

In the last section we demonstrated that change is possible, but do we have any evidence that antenatal classes are of benefit? The answer is yes. There is increasing evidence not only that women find that attendance satisfies some of their individual needs, but also that studies are more convincingly demonstrating tangible benefits.

In one of the few recently published studies on the views of the consumer, Combes and Schonveld (1992) set out to discuss with groups of pregnant women and first-time parents their experiences, feelings and concerns about becoming a parent. The study was based on 58 parents who took part in nine different discussion groups. One of these was for men only, the others were of pregnant women or first time mothers.

The results showed that most women who attended antenatal classes were positive about the experience, but, according to Combes and Schonveld, most bemoaned the lack of time to talk about individual concerns. Women did, however, enjoy the social contact with other women at the classes. Some felt that the breathing and relaxation exercises had helped their labour, and most had enjoyed the visit to the labour ward.

One difficulty with this research is that the results are not presented numerically. The only figure we are given is that of one woman who described a huge evening class she had gone to where she could hardly hear because of the numbers there. Not surprisingly, most women preferred small groups. It is difficult to judge, therefore, how widespread were the feelings expressed.

One noteworthy finding was that some women felt that 'difficult' topics, such as abnormal labour, were avoided or dealt with only briefly. They felt that the teachers tended to dismiss anxieties or negative feelings.

A matter of some concern was the finding that advice given in the classes was often found to differ from that from other health professionals.

Interestingly, there was a complaint that in some classes very little time was given to considering what happens after the birth and how to cope with being a parent. For first time mothers, this was a common and important criticism. Some women commented that the classes focused too much on the baby and not enough on the feelings and experiences of the mother.

The strength of this study design was that it included those who had not gone to any classes. Amongst this group, it was found that most felt that they did not need to attend. They were happy with the information they already had, and many mentioned having found out a lot from friends and family. An important finding was that some single women did not go to classes because they associated them with failing to cope. They felt confident about their pregnancies and were particularly anxious to be seen to be coping well, especially as they knew that health professionals were often very concerned about single parents.

Overall, this study reinforces earlier research and illustrates that there are many issues previously identified that have still not been adequately addressed. The results show that benefits are possible, particularly where groups are small and the sessions take account of individual need.

Is it possible to find more tangible benefits from attending antenatal classes? This was the aim of Simkin and Enkin's (1989) review of the literature on classes. In their conclusion, based on an exhaustive review of the more 'scientific' research on the subject, they say that an evaluation of the effectiveness of antenatal classes is not easy. This is due to the difficulty of designing and conducting well-controlled trials.

They also point out that the attitudes conveyed in classes, the quality of the instruction and the specific techniques taught all vary. This makes it impossible to generalise about the effects of antenatal classes per se. Evaluation is further complicated by the difficulty of separating the question of whether the skills taught in the classes can work if appropriately used, from whether or not women actually use (or even have the opportunity to use) the skills they are taught.

Simkin and Enkin make two important points concerning evaluation. First, the effectiveness of an individual teacher or class programme is unquestionably one factor in determining the effectiveness of antenatal classes in any particular setting. Second, Simkin and Enkin draw attention to the important variable of the support received during labour, both from the professionals and from a supportive partner. This could have the effect of enhancing the preparation given at classes, but it could also override poor teaching or indeed inhibit the preparation that has been given. They comment that both effective teaching and consistent follow-up in labour, encouraging the use of the learned strategies, is required to ensure that women can indeed use what they have learned.

However, the authors reveal that the existing evidence suggests that women who attend antenatal classes use less analgesic medication and feel less pain in labour, although pain levels can still be very high. They point out that the wide variation in results from different studies may depend not only on differences in the classes, but also on the support provided by the caregivers in labour. Simkin and Enkin end by warning that the possible adverse effects of antenatal classes have not been systematically evaluated; the very existence of classes and their growing popularity appear to have contributed to significant changes in maternity care – presumably they mean for the better.

One of the most important new studies that has attempted to test whether some of the aims of antenatal classes are achieved is a British study by Hillier and Slade (1989). This looked at the effect of antenatal class attendance on knowledge, anxiety and confidence in primiparous women. A further aim was to compare community with hospital-based classes.

The authors attempted to avoid some of the pitfalls of previous studies by using before and after measurements with the same individuals, and by making assessments immediately before and on completion of the classes, rather than some time later. They also used a knowledge scale whose reliability had been tested and shown to be accurate. The sample consisted of 31 women attending hospital-based classes and 36 in the community. Importantly, the format and content of the classes were very similar.

Taking the two groups of women together, they found that there was a significant increase in knowledge following classes, with average scores rising from 54 to 75 per cent. Ten out of the 12 questions on the test questionnaire showed significant increases in the scores achieved. Their conclusion was that the greatest potential for further learning relates to questions concerning diet, the role of the second stage of labour, smoking and the benefits of breastfeeding.

The results on anxiety levels showed that there was a reduction in the trait anxiety levels of the sample, that is, anxiety relating to the individual rather than the situation. It was also found that there were highly significant increases in confidence concerning labour and caring for the newborn child. Their conclusion based on these findings was that knowledge and confidence levels showed substantial increases over the period of the classes.

Unfortunately, as the design did not include a non-attending control group, it is impossible to say that the results have been produced by the attendance at the classes. It could be that the increase in knowledge and confidence might have happened anyway, without attending classes.

Comparing the two locations of classes, it was found that community classes were equally as effective in communicating knowledge and improving confidence as were hospital-based classes. However, they had the additional benefit that more women developed friendships amongst others attending. As there is growing evidence in the literature that social support may be a protective factor against depression following delivery, the authors suggest that this is a strong argument in support of community-based classes.

☐ **Improving classes**

How can we improve classes? The following suggestions come from Combes and Schonveld (1992) and appear to include most of the issues that have been covered so far in this review. They suggest that there should be:

- More emphasis on childcare and living with a new baby, including teaching care skills;

- More emphasis on the role of a parent, including social and psychological adjustments;

- Acknowledgement of negative as well as positive feelings and experiences, both in pregnancy and after the birth;

- Use of the experiences of a newly delivered mother to help women increase their understanding of the postnatal period;

- More information about labour complications and what can go wrong;

- Promotion of realistic expectations of labour pain levels and of the postnatal period;

- More emphasis on the role of partners in labour and of the father's role during pregnancy and after the birth;

- An equal emphasis given to the needs and experiences of the parent and the baby;

- A greater emphasis on the social, emotional and psychological aspects of pregnancy and parenting.

(Combes and Schonveld 1992: 35)

■ Health promotion

So far the emphasis has been on health education in the form of antenatal classes, but this is not the only form that parent education takes. Throughout their contacts with women, midwives are constantly engaging in health education activities. In addition, in recent years, there has been a new focus of attention in the form of health promotion. In this section, the issue of the midwife's role in health promotion will be examined.

As with classes, we must first of all identify the aim of health promotion and ask whether there is sufficient evidence to justify midwifery involvement. If there is such evidence, on what aspects should this activity focus?

□ **Defining health promotion**

A number of writers have pointed out that there is confusion over the exact meaning of health promotion and how it differs from health education (Ewles & Simnett 1992; Tones & Tilford 1994; Webb 1994). Over 10 years ago, Tannahill (1985) stated that health promotion is a highly fashionable term that has acquired so many meanings as to become meaningless. Furthermore, he pointed out, it is one of those terms that people tend to throw around glibly, without spelling out their interpretations. The same view is expressed by Ewles and Simnett (1992), who suggest that there is currently no clear, widely adopted consensus on what is meant by health promotion.

If we look at the origins of the concept, we find that although the term health promotion is credited as first used by the Canadian health minister, Marc Lalonde, in 1974 (Naidoo & Wills 1994), the most frequently used description is that produced by the World Health Organization (WHO) in what has become known as the Ottawa Charter (WHO 1986). In this, health promotion was defined as 'enabling people to increase control over, and improve their health'. The following were offered as the essential elements of a policy aimed at health promotion:

1. Building a healthy public policy
2. Creating supportive environments
3. Developing personal skills
4. Strengthening community action
5. Reorienting health services

(WHO 1986: 1)

From this, we can see that health promotion is a far wider activity than health education. In the latter, the target is seen as the individual and changes in individual lifestyle and behaviour related to health. In health promotion, although individuals are still important, there is a recognition that there are other influences on health, including environmental, political and social factors.

The two concepts of health education and health promotion are brought together by the WHO (1986) when they say that health promotion programmes are designed to promote health and that health education will be an integral part of that activity. This has led Ewles and Simnett (1992) to suggest the use of health promotion as an umbrella term for a range of activities including health education.

This has been further clarified by Naidoo and Wills (1994), who make the point that the process of attempting to promote health may include a whole range of interventions including:

- those which foster healthy lifestyles
- those which encourage access to services and involvement in health decisions
- those which seek to promote an environment in which the healthy choice becomes the easier choice
- those which educate about the body and keeping healthy

(Naidoo and Wills 1994: 62)

All of these seem to describe the activities of the midwife in formal and informal settings in all their contacts with women and their families.

☐ **The argument for midwifery involvement in health promotion**

Should health promotion be acknowledged as an integral part of midwifery activities, or is it a service luxury? There are two answers to this question; the first comes from government reports and the second from evidence on its success.

The importance of health promotion has been made clear from government reports such as *The strategy for nursing* (DoH 1989), which contains the following recommendation:

Health education and health promotion should be a recognised part of health care; all practitioners should develop skills in, and use every opportunity for, health promotion.

(DoH 1989: 32)

More recently, the *Health of the nation* report (DoH 1992) has predicted that over the next 10 years, health gains will increasingly depend on action in health promotion and disease prevention.

The conclusion from these government reports is that health promotion must be seen as essential to midwifery activity. However, we must still determine whether time spent on this activity will be productive.

In answer to the question 'Does health promotion work?', Naidoo and Wills (1994) state that the overwhelming weight of evidence is that health promotion in general does work. They cite three studies that looked at published reports of health promotion interventions and found that all three concluded that the majority of health promotion interventions are effective. One review of health promotion they cite found that 85 per cent of 62 studies reported improved knowledge levels, 65 per cent of 39 studies reported improved attitudes in the desired direction, and 75 per cent of 123 studies reported behavioural change.

Although this is reassuring, it leaves a number of studies that were unable to demonstrate clear advantages. Garcia *et al* (1994), in the summary of their review of published evidence relating to health promotion and infant health, are more cautious about the evidence on effectiveness. Although they conclude that there is potential for improving health outcomes for babies, they say that, so far, few studies of health promotion interventions have shown reliably that reductions in mortality or major morbidity can be achieved. They do go on to admit, however, that the recent striking fall in the rate of cot deaths may prove to be an exception to this.

The evidence is therefore mixed. This does not necessarily mean that health promotion does not work, but, as Garcia *et al* suggest, it may mean that the methods of evaluating some of the interventions may suffer from flaws that are unable to demonstrate the success of the interventions. It could also suggest that studies have been unable to limit the influence of other factors that may have played a part in the outcomes.

□   **The main targets of health promotion**

If we accept that health promotion activities are worth pursuing, what should midwives target? Here there is more consensus on the areas that should be considered. The following are suggested by Roch (1992: 14) as key areas in which midwives could have considerable impact if patterns of practice were slightly modified or extended:

- Preconception care;
- Eating and drinking habits (including food safety);
- Smoking;
- Communicable diseases;
- Prevention of accidents;
- Neonatal care.

Interestingly, this is mainly a list of behavioural factors that have physical consequences. Outcomes such as postnatal depression or difficulties with social readjustments associated with a change in social role are not highlighted, although they are briefly mentioned in Hillan (1994).

An additional topic that may become more important is information on HIV/AIDS (Roth & Brierley 1990; Roth 1995). According to Roth and Brierley (1990), midwives meet all women who attend for antenatal care and are often in the privileged position of learning about a woman's lifestyle and concerns about her sexual life. This places midwives in a particularly favourable position to inform and educate about the sexual spread of HIV and, if it is relevant, the hazards of shared needles and syringes.

☐ **Implications for the midwife**

The acceptance of health promotion activities as part of midwifery activities will inevitably have a number of implications. The skills required to undertake this activity is an obvious issue that will need to be addressed. Garcia *et al* (1994) also point out that changing lifestyles requires a great deal of commitment from those who are being asked to make the change. It is therefore necessary that advice is not only based on sound evidence, but is also imparted in ways that give women the incentive to make the required effort.

The issue of how information is provided has also been highlighted by Naidoo and Wills (1994), who warn that respecting clients' autonomy can be difficult for health promoters. There is often a tendency, they suggest, to neglect the autonomy of the individual and to give advice, to offer information or to persuade clients to change their behaviour. The challenge, then, is to accept the role of partner and enabler rather than of expert and controller. This danger of taking over from the client is also identified by Ewles and Simnett (1992), who list three common ways in which health promoters hinder rather than respect their client's autonomy:

- By imposing their own solutions to the client's problems

- By instructing clients on what to do because s/he takes too long to work it out for him or herself

- By dismissing the client's ideas without providing an adequate explanation or the opportunity to try them out

(Ewles & Simnett 1992: 122)

It is clear that entering into the arena of health promotion requires considerable skills on the part of the midwife and a clear strategy on the part of midwifery services.

This was also the conclusion of a workshop on health promotion for senior and experienced representatives of nursing, midwifery and health visiting practice reported by Parish *et al* (1991). There was unanimity among the participants that staff do not possess all the knowledge and skills necessary to undertake the role of health promoter. Basic counselling and advocacy skills were seen as essential prerequisites for health promotion. The workshop also concluded that an education strategy was crucial in developing the health promotion role of nurses, midwives and health visitors for the future.

Since that workshop, a great deal has been written on health promotion, and a number of courses are now available to ensure that midwives develop a broad understanding of relevant theories and approaches. It is appropriate to end with one example of guidelines that have been produced on the basis of research evidence.

Naidoo and Wills (1994) point out that the evidence from people who have changed their health behaviour suggests that there are certain minimum conditions required for that change to take place. They list these as including the following:

- the change must be self-initiated

- the behaviour must become salient, that is an issue rather than something that happens almost without thought

- the salience of the behaviour must appear over a period of time

- the behaviour should not be part of the individual's coping strategies

- the individual's life should not be problematic or uncertain – there is a limit to a person's capacity to adapt and change. For example, those living on a low income will be stretched by coping with poverty and its uncertainties. Having to make changes in their health behaviour may be too much to expect for people whose lives are already problematic

- social support must be available

(Naidoo & Wills 1994: 193)

These are important points if the midwife is to apply the principles of health promotion in a sensitive and professional way that is research based and that realises that it may not be possible or desirable to implement health promotion in every case.

■ Recommendations for clinical practice in the light of currently available evidence

There is sufficient evidence to support the continued use of antenatal classes as a worthwhile and cost effective part of midwifery services. However, if the full potential is to be achieved, there are a number of suggestions based on the research evidence that should be considered.

1. The aim of classes should be redefined to ensure that they take account of current philosophies, for example empowerment and informed choice.

2. Sessions should be run, as far as possible, using participatory learning approaches.

3. Staff involved in the classes should be trained in group skills methods and should have a flair for this approach to teaching. Above all, they should want to be involved in classes.

4. Community classes should be acknowledged as having the additional benefits of facilitating friendships, which may play a part in reducing levels of postnatal depression.

5. The needs of partners and their attendance at antenatal sessions should be considered as part of service provision.

It is also important that midwifery considers the wider aspect of health promotion, which can be incorporated into activities throughout pregnancy and the puerperium. In relation to this, a number of additional recommendations can be made.

6. Midwives should receive appropriate education to allow them to carry out health promotion. This should include counselling and advocacy skills.

7. Health promotional activities should be based on sound research knowledge.

8. Local strategies on health promotion should be developed, and these should be linked with the involvement of other relevant health professional groups.

■ Practice check

For those involved in antenatal sessions, it is important to consider a number of aspects regarding these sessions.

● Is the content influenced by, and based on, the needs of attenders?

● Are sessions conducted in an environment that encourages questions, queries and comments?

● Do the sessions provide information that will allow informed choices to be made?

For those involved in health promotional activities, the following additional questions should be posed.

- Am I clear on the meaning and scope of health promotion?
- Have I identified the potential areas for health promotion in my activities?
- Am I aware of those topics that have been demonstrated to be effective in terms of outcomes?
- Am I conversant with the alternative approaches to health promotion and the consequences of the approach I use in terms of its likely effect on those receiving it?
- Is it possible that my current approach may actually have a negative affect?
- Is there a local strategy for health promotion?

■ References

Clements J 1989 Antenatal education. Nursing Standard   4(10): 51–4

Cogan G 1983 Variations in the effectiveness of childbirth preparation. Perinatal Press   7(4): 51–4

Combes G, Schonveld 1992 Life will never be the same again – learning to be a first-time parent: a review of antenatal and post-natal health education. Health Education Authority, London

Davies C 1989 High hopes. Nursing Times Community Outlook Supplement August: 15

Department of Health 1989 The strategy for nursing. London, HMSO

Department of Health 1992 The health of the nation. London, HMSO

Dunwoody M, Watters P 1990 Becoming a mother. Health Visitor   63(10): 335–8

Ewles L, Simnett I 1992 Promoting health, 2nd edn. John Wiley, Chichester

Garcia J, France-Dawson M, Macfarlane A 1994 Improving infant health. The effectiveness of health promotion activities to reduce still birth, infant mortality and morbidity: a literature review. Health Education Authority, London

Gilkison A 1991 Antenatal education – whose purposes does it serve? New Zealand College of Midwives Journal   4: 13–15 (also published in MIDIRS Midwifery Digest 1991   1[4]: 418–20)

Hillan E 1994 The mother and baby. In Webb P (ed.) Health promotion and patient education. A professional's guide. Chapman & Hall, London, p59–79

Hillier C, Slade P 1989 The impact of antenatal classes on knowledge, anxiety and confidence in primiparous women. Journal of Reproductive and Infant Psychology   7(1): 3–13

Murphy-Black T 1990 Antenatal education. In Alexander J, Levy V, Roch S (eds) Antenatal care: a research-based approach. Macmillan, Basingstoke, Ch 6, p88–104

Murphy-Black T, Faulkner A (eds) 1988 Antenatal group skills training. A manual of guidelines. John Wiley, Chichester

Naidoo J, Wills J 1994 Health promotion: foundations for practice. Baillière Tindall, Eastbourne

O'Connor Y 1993 Education for parenthood: a time for change! Midwives Chronicle 106(1265): 198–201

Parish R, Powell C, Wilkes E 1991 Health promotion in nursing practice. Nursing Standard 5(23): 37–40

Perkins E 1978 Having a baby: an educational experience? Leverhume Health Education Project. Occasional Paper No 6. University of Nottingham, Nottingham.

Perkins E 1979 Preparation for parenthood. A critique of the concept. Leverhume Health Education Project. Occasional Paper No 17. University of Nottingham, Nottingham

Perkins E 1980 Education for childbirth and parenthood. Croom Helm, London

Priest J, Schott J 1991 Leading antenatal classes: a practical guide. Butterworth–Heinemann, Oxford

Rees C 1982 Antenatal classes: time for a new approach. Nursing Times 78(48): 1446–8

Rees C 1993 Antenatal classes: has midwifery lost interest? British Journal of Midwifery 1(2): 75–7

Roch S 1992 Client wants and needs. Modern Midwife 2(2): 14–15

Roth C (1995) HIV and pregnancy. In Alexander J, Levy V, Roch S (eds) Aspects of midwifery practice: a research-based approach. Macmillan, Basingstoke, Ch 6, p109–31

Roth C, Brierley J 1990 HIV infection – a midwifery perspective. In Alexander J, Levy V, Roch S (eds) Intrapartum care: a research-based approach. Macmillan, Basingstoke, p154–72

Simkin P, Enkin M 1989 Antenatal classes. In Chalmers I, Enkin M, Keirse M (eds) Effective care in pregnancy. Oxford University Press, Oxford, p318–34

Tannahill A 1985 What is health promotion? Health Education Journal 44(4): 167–8

Tones K, Tilford S 1994 Health education: effectiveness, efficiency and equity, 2nd edn. Chapman & Hall, London

Turner S 1993 How to enjoy teaching parentcraft classes. Midwives Chronicle 106(1265): 210–15

Webb P 1994 Some ethical issues in health and patient education. In Webb P (ed.) Health promotion and patient education. A professional's guide. Chapman & Hall, London, p38–56

World Health Organization 1986 Ottawa charter for health promotion. An international conference on health promotion, 17–21 November 1986. WHO regional office for Europe, Copenhagen

Chapter 5

Fetal wellbeing: the intrauterine environment and ensuing legal and ethical issues

Elsa Montgomery

Beliefs about the effects of the intrauterine *milieu* on fetal wellbeing have been in existence since ancient times. These have ranged from concerns that a pregnant woman should be surrounded by beautiful objects to the need to avoid intoxicating substances.

Ideas about what might cause harm have changed over the years and continue to do so. This is evidenced by the thalidomide tragedy of the 1960s. In just the past 5 years, warnings about listeria contamination of certain foods have been issued in England. Now attention is focused on the ramifications of fetal wellbeing not only for the neonatal period, but also in the long term, with implications for adult health and disease.

Obviously, this is an all-embracing subject. Discussions in this chapter are necessarily limited and encompass alcohol (concentrating on 'moderate' consumption), smoking (especially passive smoking) and effects on long-term health. The chapter ends with a consideration of legal and ethical issues.

■ **It is assumed that you are already aware of the following:**

● The features of fetal alcohol syndrome;

● What constitutes 1 unit of alcohol;

● The physiological effects of smoking on mother and baby;

- The grounds for termination of pregnancy as set out in the Abortion Act 1967 (amended by the Human Fertilisation and Embryology Act 1990);

- The basic contents of the Congenital Disability (Civil Liability) Act 1976.

■ Alcohol

Since fetal alcohol syndrome was first recognised and named in the early 1970s, the body of evidence showing effects of heavy alcohol consumption in pregnancy (that is, at levels at which the mother is likely to have problems with alcohol abuse) has grown. While there is little doubt that alcohol intake at such levels can have a major deleterious effect on the fetus, it has been more difficult to clarify the situation with regards to 'social' drinking. In her chapter on 'Maternal alcohol and tobacco use during pregnancy' for the first volume in this series, Moira Plant (1990) found that debate continued on whether or not pregnant women should abstain from drinking alcohol altogether. To what extent has this issue been resolved in the past 5 years?

□ Moderate alcohol consumption in pregnancy

Mills *et al* (1984) conducted one of the largest studies attempting to ascertain a safe level for drinking in pregnancy. They designed a large-scale prospective cohort study, collecting data by questionnaire from a sample of 34 660 pregnant women attending clinics for their first visit. Thus their information was limited to alcohol use during the first trimester. Women were asked to estimate their daily alcohol consumption (six or more, three to five, one or two, or less than one drink per day). Each woman's medical records were also reviewed. Birthweights and odds ratios for being small for gestational age were adjusted for possible confounding factors. They discovered a reduction in birthweight with increasing alcohol consumption, except amongst the heaviest drinkers, who were few in number. Compared with non-drinkers, babies of the lightest drinkers showed a mean reduction of 14 g in birthweight, while those consuming three to five drinks per day were 165 g lighter.

The risk of producing a baby below the tenth centile for weight at each level of drinking, compared to abstainers, is shown in Table 5.1. Thus for those who had only an occasional drink, the effect on birthweight was trivial, and the risks of producing a low birthweight or small-for-gestational-age baby was only slightly higher than that for non-drinkers. However, the authors describe a substantial increase in risk

Table 5.1 Odds ratios for a small-for-gestational-age* birth by alcohol
consumption adjusted by multiple logistic regression (reproduced from Mills *et al*
1984, with permission)

Variable No. of drinks per day	Odds ratios†	95% Confidence intervals	*p* value
≤ 1	1.11	1.00 to 1.23	.05
1–2	1.62	1.26 to 2.09	.0002
3–5	1.96	1.16 to 3.31	.01
≥ 6	2.28	0.91 to 5.77	.08

* Less than tenth percentile for sex, race and gestational age.
† Compared with non-drinkers.

where at least one to two drinks are consumed each day, and for heavy
drinkers the risk is approximately twice that of non-drinkers.

Certain potential sources of bias need to be noted. First, information was
only gathered on the first trimester, which does not allow for changing
habits once pregnancy was confirmed or after being specifically asked on
the subject in the questionnaire. Because women were asked about average
drinking, the effect of binges cannot be ascertained.

Virji (1991) looked at patterns of alcohol consumption in 5400
women from an American National Natality Survey. Data were collected
retrospectively after birth. Women were asked how often they drank and
how many drinks they would have on days when alcohol was taken. A
Quality–Frequency Index of alcohol intake was calculated. The heaviest
drinking group was defined as that taking two or more drinks per day –
very different from the six or more categorized by Mills *et al*.

Confirming the results of Mills *et al*, a dose–response relationship
emerged, the percentage of low birthweight infants increasing as levels of
alcohol increased. However, while the first study identified a mean reduction in birthweight of 165 g for those consuming three to five drinks per
day, Virji recorded a difference of 487 g between 'heavy' drinkers and
abstainers. The percentage of low birthweight babies born within each
drinking category was also greater, but this seems to reflect a higher incidence of low birthweight generally in the study. Virji found that 14
per cent of abstainers had low birthweight infants, compared with 4 per
cent in the study by Mills *et al*. In the latter study, 24.2 per cent of newborns whose mothers consumed three or more drinks a day weighed less
than 2500 g, compared with 33 per cent in the former, where mothers
took more than two alcoholic drinks per day.

By contrast, in a much smaller study, Zaluska *et al* (1993) apparently
found no direct relationship between birthweight and alcohol. However,
they defined heavy drinking as more than one drink a *month* and moderate drinking as less than this. It is questionable how useful results based

on such categories can be, especially as 'heavy drinkers' accounted for only 4.6 per cent of the sample (23 out of 495).

Tolo and Little (1993) looked specifically at the effect of occasional binges by moderate drinkers. Data about the month before conception and the first two trimesters of pregnancy were collected by a self-administered questionnaire from 5298 pregnant members of a US health insurance-related organisation. Moderate drinking was defined as less than two drinks per day before pregnancy and less than one per day during pregnancy. A 'binge' was defined as at least five drinks on one occasion. This was a well-motivated population, and the mean average alcohol consumption for women who binged and for those who did not was less than one drink per week during pregnancy. No adverse fetal outcome with regards to birthweight, gestational age or Apgar score could be found.

☐ **Effects on development**

Whereas moderate alcohol intake (up to two drinks per day) appears adversely to affect birthweight, the same cannot be said for its effect on neurological development. Walpole *et al* (1991) conducted a prospective population–based cohort study of mothers who drank socially, to evaluate their offspring for various characteristics, including neurobehavioural responses. A questionnaire was completed by the 2002 women who were recruited. Of these, a subsample of 665 was chosen from a wide spectrum of drinkers, stratified by alcohol intake before pregnancy. Daily intake for group one was less than 2.8 ml of absolute alcohol, for group two was 2.8–27.9 ml (that is, up to approximately two drinks) and for group three was more than 28 ml. No significant association between low-to-moderate maternal alcohol intake (this level not being quantified by the authors) and neonatal behaviour was found except for an unspecified 'minimal effect' on muscle tone. This was not thought likely to be of functional significance.

Forrest *et al* (1991) aimed to determine the nature of the relationship between maternal alcohol consumption before, during and after pregnancy with infant mental and motor development at 18 months of age. They followed up children born to 846 primigravidae in Dundee between May 1985 and April 1986. Alcohol consumption was calculated as an average amount of absolute alcohol in grams consumed weekly. Various confounding factors were taken into account. All the children were assessed by a trained psychologist, who was blind to knowledge of maternal drinking.

Scores achieved by the infants gave a mental development index and a psychomotor index. The former was positively related to social class but not to alcohol consumption – although alcohol consumption was higher among the lower social classes. There was little relation between the latter and social class and none with alcohol consumption.

☐ **Alcohol and risks of spontaneous abortion**

A further concern expressed about alcohol consumption in pregnancy is the possibility of increased risk of miscarriage. Studies performed to examine this issue have shown conflicting results and are open to certain criticisms. Parazzini *et al* (1990, 1994) report two similarly designed case control studies from Northern Italy. The former was small scale, involving 94 cases comprising an atypical group of women who had not had a full-term pregnancy but had suffered two or more unexplained miscarriages. The latter involved 462 women admitted to obstetric departments for spontaneous abortion in the first 12 weeks of pregnancy. The controls, numbering 176 and 814 respectively, had given birth to healthy infants at the same hospitals on randomly selected days. The first study compared three groups:

1. Non-drinkers;

2. Those consuming fewer than two drinks per day;

3. Those consuming more than two drinks per day.

The second study also used three categories: no or occasional alcohol, one to seven drinks per week, and more than seven drinks per week. Their results were fairly consistent, indicating that moderate alcohol consumption does not significantly increase the risk of miscarriage.

By contrast, the prospective study by Long *et al* (1994), comprising 3348 controls (women who booked consecutively with a singleton pregnancy and went on to deliver after 28 weeks) but only 95 cases (a separate but concurrent sample comprising women presenting with confirmed first trimester miscarriages) suggests that even light drinking in early pregnancy is associated with an increased risk of spontaneous abortion. (Table 5.2). They defined levels of drinking as follows:

● Non-drinkers;

● Light – 1–10 units per week;

● Moderate – 11–14 units per week;

● Heavy – more than 15 units per week.

It should be noted that in England and Wales, 1 unit of alcohol is equivalent to 8 g, whereas Parazzini *et al* describe 1 unit as being 12 g . The statistics presented in each of these three studies suggest that caution is required in interpreting the results. While Long *et al* show a significantly

Table 5.2 Relative risk (95 per cent confidence intervals) of spontaneous first trimester miscarriage in drinkers (*n*=3009) compared with non-drinkers (*n*=434) (reproduced from Long *et al* 1994, with permission)

	Relative risk	*n*
Light drinkers	3.79 (1.18–12.17)	2349
Moderate drinkers	8.36 (2.52–27.69)	499
Heavy drinkers	5.08 (1.18–21.84)	161

increased risk of miscarriage amongst drinkers, their confidence intervals are very wide (probably owing to the small sample of cases). By contrast, Parazzini *et al*, in both of their studies, intimate a negligible risk, and from their figures, a slightly protective effect of alcohol could equally be inferred.

As suggested earlier, there has been considerable debate over whether light or moderate drinking in pregnancy threatens fetal wellbeing. The problem is compounded by methodological difficulties. All the studies discussed here rely on self-reporting of alcohol consumption, which is likely to be subject to underestimation. Several of them were retrospective, collecting data after birth, when it is possible that knowledge of the outcome may bias recall. However, the major problem in attempting to compare research and draw conclusions is the lack of consistency in measures used or definitions of levels of drinking. Furthermore, most studies calculate average alcohol intake, which could mean a small amount each day or a large amount less often. As Knupfer (1991) points out, there is potentially a big difference between one drink each day of the week and seven drinks in one day. It is also extremely difficult to control for confounding factors. Women who drink in pregnancy tend to be older, of higher parity and unmarried, and to smoke and to consume more coffee than those who do not drink (Taylor 1993).

It has become fashionable in recent years, especially in America, to recommend total abstinence from alcohol when pregnant or planning a pregnancy (for example Committee on Substance Abuse and Committee on Children with Disabilities 1993). This inevitably causes guilt and anxiety amongst many women who have an occasional social drink. Knupfer (1991) is suspicious of a political or antifemale agenda behind such dogma, and indeed there is little evidence to support this position. The Health Education Authority (1993) advises that one or two units of alcohol once or twice a week during pregnancy is unlikely to be harmful. In light of the evidence presented here, this seems reasonable. At such levels, any reduction in birthweight will be minute and long-term effects improbable. However, it is not possible to state categorically that *any* alcohol in pregnancy is safe. It has been shown in studies using ultrasound scans that one drink will suppress fetal breathing movements for up to 3 hours (Lewis & Boylan 1979, McLeod et al 1983). There is no suggestion that this has serious implications for fetal health, but it never-theless demonstrates that, even in small quantities, alcohol can compro-mise fetal functioning.

Aaronson and Macnee (1989) highlight the need for health care pro-fessionals to be sensitive to realistic options for change. Many women will wish to avoid any alcohol in pregnancy, but to try to force such a position on all women is likely to be counterproductive and is not justi-fied by research evidence.

■ Smoking in pregnancy

Unlike the situation with drinking in pregnancy, where debate remains about potential harm with light-to-moderate intake, there is little dis-pute that smoking, at any level, causes fetal harm. It is widely accepted that maternal smoking leads to an average reduction in birthweight of approximately 200 g (Newnham 1991). Other deleterious effects include:

- Increased risk of spontaneous abortion;

- Increased perinatal mortality;

- Increased incidence of placenta praevia and abruption;

- Increased risk of sudden infant death syndrome.

All authors on the subject concur that any reduction in the number of cigarettes smoked, at any stage of pregnancy, is beneficial and should be encouraged. (For a review, see Aaronson & Macnee 1989; Newnham 1991; and Gillies & Wakefield 1993.)

□ Passive smoking

Less clear, but the subject of increasing interest, is the effect of exposure of non-smokers to environmental tobacco smoke.

As with studies into low levels of alcohol consumption, research is confounded by difficulties in establishing exposure. It relies on subjective measurements such as intensity of smoke, length of exposure (often with-out considering the number of people smoking at any one time, proximity to the pregnant woman, strength of cigarettes involved, and so on) or self-reporting of the number of cigarettes smoked in the company of the subject. There seems to be a general, if guarded, agreement that passive smoking has a small but nevertheless detrimental effect on birth-weight.

Mathai *et al* (1992) reported that babies born to passive smokers weighed on average 63 g less, after adjusting for other factors known to affect birthweight, than those not exposed to tobacco smoke. A dose–response relation could not be calculated as the women involved were unable to quantify their exposure. The study involved 994 women, none of whom used tobacco themselves in any form. Fifty-two per cent of them lived with smokers. Exposure outside the home was not quantified. Similarly, Zhang and Ratcliffe (1993) studied a population in which smoking amongst women was very rare but where 57 per cent of men aged 20–39 years smoked. Their data came from Shanghai Birth Defects and Perinatal Death monitoring conducted between October 1986 and September 1987 and involved 1785 non-smoking mothers. A mean decrease of 30 g in birthweight was found amongst infants exposed to environmental tobacco smoke (defined as exposure to paternal smoking). Strangely, although paternal smoking of up to 19 cigarettes a day was associated with a progressive decrease in birthweight, there appeared to be a slight increase, of 32 g, when exposed to 20 or more cigarettes a day. It is difficult to explain this as the numbers involved are not particularly small. The authors put forward some suggestions, but it is likely that it is due to a chance aberration.

Fortier *et al* (1994) looked not at birthweight *per se* but at the risk of delivering a small-for-gestational-age baby. Rather than concentrating on exposure to tobacco smoke at home, they looked also at the workplace and controlled for many confounding factors, including selected job characteristics. Data were collected by standard questionnaire over the telephone, and the sample numbered 4644 women. Passive smoking at home was not found to be related to delivering a baby small for gestational age. Overall, there was little or no higher risk when comparing those exposed to tobacco smoke and those not exposed. None of the trends was statistically significant, but where women were exposed at work, the chances of delivering a small baby were slightly greater. The risk grew with increasing number of hours worked, increasing number of weeks of exposure and increasing subjective estimation of the intensity of the smoke. These results cannot be directly compared with the above studies as the actual differences in birthweight are not reported.

Ogawa *et al* (1991) also looked at passive smoking both at home and work. Interestingly, they discovered that 30 per cent of the women with husbands who smoked daily reported no passive smoking and that 13 per cent with non-smoking husbands were exposed to tobacco smoke at home. They suggest therefore that paternal smoking habit may be an inadequate index of maternal passive exposure. A small statistically significant reduction in birthweight was seen with passive smoking, but this was eliminated by adjustment for confounding factors. The authors suggest that this crude effect is explained by the fact that the passive smokers in their sample tended to be younger and nulliparous. However, they expect from their results that heavy exposure to tobacco smoke induces a reduction in fetal growth.

Martinez *et al* (1994) studied 1246 newborns, 992 of whom had non-smoking mothers. There was a significant trend for birthweight to decrease with an increasing number of cigarettes smoked by the father. The 60 newborns of non-smoking mothers whose fathers smoked more than 20 cigarettes a day had a mean deficit in birthweight of 88 g. This was independent of other factors. In order to counter claims that the apparent effects of passive smoking may be due to misclassification of smoking mothers as non-smokers, levels of cotinine (a metabolite of nicotine) were measured in cord blood samples from 175 (14%) of the babies. All 23 subjects whose mothers smoked more than 10 cigarettes per day had detectable cotinine levels, compared with 7 (50%) of those whose mothers smoked 1–10 cigarettes a day. Cotinine was undetectable in 130 (94%) of those whose mothers were non-smokers. A further 6 (4.4%) had serum cotinine levels at the lower limit of detectability. Two babies (1.5%) of apparent non-smokers had serum cotinine concentrations clearly within the range found among the infants of active smokers. This therefore indicates that just two mothers under-reported their smoking habits. Amongst babies of non-smoking mothers, the concentration of cotinine in cord blood was strongly related to the number of cigarettes smoked by the father. The numbers here are small. Three out of 20 newborns (15%) of non-smoking mothers and smoking fathers had detectable serum cotinine. However, it was found in only 3 out of 110 newborns (2.7%) where both parents were non-smokers. It is a pity that cord cotinine was not measured on a larger proportion of the sample.

Obviously, passive smoking is less of a health issue than active smoking, and it does not appear to be a significant factor in actual growth retardation. However, it does cause a small reduction in birthweight, which, while probably not important on an individual basis, could have wider consequences across a whole population (Zhang & Ratcliffe 1993). Martinez *et al* (1994) point out that the inverse correlations between birthweight and neonatal and postneonatal mortality are not limited to low birthweight infants, and thus passive smoking by a mother may have adverse implications for her child's health during the first year of life.

■ **Fetal wellbeing and long-term health**

Factors such as smoking and drinking can be seen to have an immediate and tangible effect on the health of the infant. In recent years, there has been increasing interest in the idea that long-term health may be influenced by life *in utero*. This makes pregnancy a daunting prospect for both the mother and the midwife. In particular, in Britain, the work of

Professor Barker and colleagues links risks of mortality from various diseases to fetal and infant origins.

☐ **Fetal origins of cardiovascular disease**

Much of the work by Barker *et al* has focused on cardiovascular disease and was born from observations that large geographical differences in death rates in England and Wales remained unexplained. A paradox was noted, in that while cardiovascular disease is generally associated with affluence, the highest death rates are in the poorest parts of the country. Furthermore, there is a strong correlation between past infant mortality rates and current mortality from cardiovascular disease (Barker 1991).

It was postulated that impaired growth and development in prenatal and early postnatal life might be an important risk factor for ischaemic heart disease (Barker *et al* 1989b). This hypothesis was investigated by studying death rates in men born in Hertfordshire from 1911 to 1930, whose weights at birth and one year of age were recorded. Standard mortality ratios for ischaemic heart disease fell steeply with increasing weight at 1 year old. The overall death rate for this condition was below the national average. Those who weighed less than 5.5 lb at birth had the highest standard mortality ratio for ischaemic heart disease, at 104 (national average 100). Where birthweight was less than 5.5 lb and weight at 1 year old was less than 18 lb, the standard mortality ratio was 220. The authors argue that this was not likely to be due to continuing adverse environmental conditions, as social class at death was not related to birthweight. Thus it was seen that the observations made on geographical links between infant mortality and deaths from ischaemic heart disease were true on an individual basis.

It has been suggested that blood pressure may be a link between the intrauterine environment and the risk of cardiovascular disease (Barker et al 1989a). The relationships between blood pressure, pulse rate and intrauterine influences were examined by Barker *et al*. Data were taken from two large national samples, one of people born in 1946 (surveyed at the age of 36) and one of children born in 1970 (surveyed at the age of 10). Systolic blood pressure was found to be inversely related to birthweight in both groups. This was independent of current weight. It was also independent of gestational age and was therefore said to be attributable to fetal growth. The differences were, however, small. Amongst the 10-year-olds, mean systolic pressure in boys fell by approximately 0.38 mmHg from the lowest to the highest birthweight. In girls, the fall was 1.32 mmHg. Amongst the 36-year-olds, mean systolic pressure fell by 2.57 mmHg from the lowest to the highest birthweight in men, the fall being 1.83 mmHg for women. There was no similar trend for diastolic pressure in either group. The authors suggest this is because the range of diastolic pressures was smaller, and as measurements tended to be rounded to the nearest 10 mmHg, the effect on diastolic recordings was therefore greater.

In another study, Barker *et al* (1990) looked at blood pressure at approximately 50 years of age in 449 people born in Preston for whom measurements at birth were recorded in detail. Systolic and diastolic blood pressures were strongly linked to birthweight and placental size. The people most at risk of hypertension were those who had been small babies with large placentae. Those with the lowest blood pressures were large babies with small placentae. For each birthweight, systolic and diastolic blood pressures rose with placental weight, and for each placental weight, both pressures fell with increasing birthweight. The relation of birthweight and placental weight to blood pressure was independent of known confounding factors. The authors conclude that 'two routine measurements taken at birth were better predictors of blood pressure than any current measurement' (Barker *et al* 1990: 261).

In a study designed to test whether this relationship exists in children today, singleton children who had been born in Salisbury hospital between July 1984 and February 1985 were followed up at the age of 4 (Law *et al* 1991). Again, systolic blood pressure was found to be positively related to placental weight and inversely related to birthweight. There was seen to be an association with restricted fetal growth and systolic blood pressure. The highest systolic blood pressures were found in children who were small babies with big placentae. However, the magnitude of the relation was less than in the study of adults and at the margins of significance. The authors suggest that it therefore needs verification.

In a review article on fetal nutrition and cardiovascular disease in adult life, Barker *et al* (1993) discuss in some detail the association between early growth patterns and disease in adults. They submit that fetal nutrition, as determined by the intrauterine environment, is the main influence on fetal growth. It is suggested that the adaptations made by the fetus, in order to survive undernutrition, permanently change the body's physiology, structure and metabolism and may lead to cardiovascular disease later in life.

☐ **Criticisms**

As suggested by Elford *et al*, the possibility that experiences in early life influence the subsequent risk of cardiovascular disease 'excites the imagination' (Elford *et al* 1991: 1). It is, however, important to be aware of the limitations incumbent upon research spanning several decades and relying heavily on retrospective data. Several of the studies involved employ ecological methods, which, Elford *et al* contend, serve to generate rather than test hypotheses. In two review articles, they question the existence of a causal link in any of the research yet conducted into the long-term implications of fetal wellbeing. They suggest that where links appear to exist, they could equally be due to persisting nutritional and socio-economic conditions, rather than to any sort of early 'programming' (Elford *et al* 1991, 1992).

This latter possibility is also highlighted by Robinson (1992), who indicates further difficulties associated with the indirectness of the methods used. It is patent that those who died as infants cannot be studied as adults and thus proxies are involved, for instance, past infant mortality as a proxy for circumstances affecting the fetus and infant, and past maternal mortality as a proxy for poor maternal health and nutrition. However, Robinson contends that the effects are really due to 'program-ming' at critical early periods and gives reasons for believing this to be so. He identifies very strong relationships, for example between birth-weight, placental weight and blood pressure, which are graded (that is, blood pressure increases progressively as birthweight decreases). These are also very specific – not all indicators of early disadvantage cause all diseases of interest. In studies of living people, risks were independent of socioeconomic factors either current or at birth. Robinson also suggests that the programming hypothesis is both plausible and biologically feasible and points to evidence from animal studies in corroboration.

These studies probably beg as many question as they answer, but their implications are awe-inspiring. As stated by Barker (1991, p132):

> We can reasonably suspect that the seeds of ill health in the next century are being sown today wherever girls and mothers have nutritional deficiencies whose nature we do not yet know.

■ Legal and ethical implications

The burden of responsibility on a mother-to-be is substantial. It would appear that at stake is not only the wellbeing of her baby, but also that of future generations. The potential for conflict between her interests and those of the fetus is therefore considerable. By their very nature, ethical conflicts cannot be resolved to the satisfaction of everyone. Arguments are often constructed on the basis of premises that others would not hold. As such, no answers are to be found in this section, merely a discussion of the issues involved.

□ The nature of the conflict

The extent to which a mother can be compelled to change her lifestyle or undergo procedures against her wishes for the sake of her unborn child is the subject of much debate.

The fact that the antenatal environment is accepted as being of considerable importance to the development of the fetus and child is evidenced by the provision of special (often free) health care and benefits to pregnant women (Sutherland 1990). Few would question the right of every child to start life in as good a state of health as possible. However, acceptance of this position requires the dilemma to be addressed of whether or not it is legitimate for society to intervene (Sutherland 1990).

As discussed by Montgomery (1994), if a person has *rights*, his or her interests justify imposing duties on others to respect or further those interests. When the rights of others are at stake, we are no longer free to pursue our own self-interest without regard for them. The critical question is whether or not a fetus has rights.

☐ **The fetus as a person**

In English law, the fetus does not have 'personality' until it is born alive (Thomson 1994). This does not mean that it has no legal protection, otherwise termination of pregnancy would be available on demand. However, the grounds for abortion indicate that the interests of the mother have primacy over those of the fetus. In the Congenital Disability (Civil Liability) Act 1976, the ability of the child to sue depends on pre-existing liability to one or other of the parents. The fetus is accorded no rights independent of them. Any rights accrue only after the fetus has been born alive (Thomson 1994). Furthermore, the child is explicitly prevented from suing its mother (except in the case of a car accident, when in practice it is the insurance company that is being sued).

However, while it may legally be possible simply to declare when the fetus becomes a person, and therefore has rights, morally the position is more difficult. A detailed discussion on the ethical standing of the fetus is beyond the scope of this chapter. Suffice it to say that, for many, it is difficult to make a distinction in status from conception to birth and beyond (Eekelaar 1988). Kennedy (1990) argues that the fetus does have rights, albeit weak, as they pertain to an entity whose fate is inextricably linked to another. He goes on to suggest that if this is so, the unborn child is owed certain duties by its mother. These include avoidance of being exposed to harm.

☐ **Implications for the mother**

To confer rights on the fetus potentially creates a position for the woman in which infringement of her basic freedom occurs. The relationship between mother and unborn child is unique as the latter has no existence independent from the former. Any attempt to control the fetal environment will inevitably impose restrictions on the woman. However, the liberty to choose what will happen to oneself is a basic precept in our society. As such 'the body constitutes the major locus of separation between the individual and the world and is in that sense the first object of each person's freedom' (Tribe, in Thomson 1994: 128). Therefore to subjugate the woman in the interests of the fetus is to render her less than an autonomous being. This has happened on at least one occasion in this country and several times in the USA.

In October 1992, the High Court declared it lawful for a hospital to perform a caesarean section on a woman against her consent. The operation was necessary owing to obstructed labour with the fetus in a transverse lie. There was said to be the gravest risk of the woman's uterus rupturing and the situation was described as 'life and death' for both mother and baby. Doctors were permitted to override the wishes of both the mother and the father, who objected on religious grounds (Thomson 1994). Sadly, the baby died before the caesarean section took place.

In America, women have been forced to undergo both caesarean sections and blood transfusions against their wishes and have been sent to prison for minor offences to protect the fetus. Thomson reports the detention of a 16-year-old for her 'tendency to be on the run' and lack of motivation or ability to seek prenatal care. In the USA, as in Britain, the fetus has no legal rights, but, as Thomson discusses, such developments illustrate 'the dangers of enforcing a state interest in the wellbeing of the fetus' (Thomson 1994: 132). Such gross denial of an individual's right to self-determination is difficult to justify. A situation can be envisaged where · a paternalistic state could impose restrictions on a mother simply because her lifestyle was not one condoned by the establishment.

For Thomson, a mother has the right to decide upon a course of action, even if it may result in harm to the fetus. This is a view also held by Kennedy, who believes it to be an uncontentious proposition that a 'woman (including a pregnant woman) has a right to autonomy, of which the right to privacy and to be free from unwanted bodily interference is one important aspect' (Kennedy 1990: 172). Not all authors would agree. Sutherland (1990) argues that where a mother proceeds with the pregnancy, it is foreseeable that certain behaviour might cause harm to the baby. For her, it is simply another example of a duty, which all people owe, not to cause harm to others. Both Sutherland (1990) and Eekelaar (1988) view pregnancy and child care as a continuum – if a mother is expected to behave reasonably towards her baby after birth, why not before? This latter argument has certain merits. Parenthood is a state involving great responsibility and, as Eekelaar points out, generally involves considerable self-denial. More weight is lent to the argument when the effect on future generations is brought into the equation.

☐ **Resolving the conflict**

While it is possible to believe that a mother is morally obliged to protect her unborn baby, it is more difficult to justify compulsion and legal enforcement. To do so would risk unpalatable restriction of women's freedom, which in turn could cause resentment towards childrearing and reluctance to seek antenatal care at all (Kennedy 1990). Sutherland (1990) recognises this but nevertheless submits that intrusion is justified in order to optimise the health of the baby and to produce individuals capable of participating fully in society.

Kennedy (1990) proposes a 'calculus' that weighs the strength of the fetus' claim against the degree of limitation or risk to the mother. This would include balancing such factors as the nature of the risk or threat to the fetus, the causal link between the conduct of the mother and the risk, the time-frame involved, the stage of development of the fetus and the degree of limitation on the woman's choice.

Difficulties arise, however, in where to draw the line. Should sanctions be imposed if a mother continues to smoke during pregnancy – or if she regularly socialises in a very smoky environment? At what level of alcohol consumption would intervention be necessary? Can a woman be forced to eat a healthy diet or cut out foods that have the potential for harm? Apart from deciding exactly what constitutes reasonable behaviour in pregnancy, a major problem is one of enforcement. There are few measures that would be effective in imposing a change in behaviour. Detention is plainly unacceptable and sanctions applied after birth are as likely to penalise the child as the parents.

Midwives obviously believe in the importance of the antenatal period, or they would not put as much energy into monitoring and education as they do. Most pregnant women feel obliged to do all they can to ensure a healthy baby and willingly forgo elements of their liberty to do so (Jones 1994). This is surely where the answer is to be found. Midwives and mothers are not adversaries but partners. Through education, advice and honest interpretation of research evidence, midwives are in an excellent position to encourage all women to accept their responsibilities.

■ **Recommendations for clinical practice in the light of currently available evidence**

1. One or two alcoholic drinks once or twice a week is probably a reasonable limit during pregnancy.

2. Women who have several drinks on one occasion before they discover they are pregnant can be reassured that it is unlikely to cause harm.

3. Pregnant women should avoid being exposed to environmental cigarette smoke regularly, but occasional exposure is not likely to have a detrimental effect.

4. Opinion varies on the justifiability of legal restrictions on pregnant women. In practice, there are few strategies that could be employed successfully. Therefore, the onus rests on the midwife and other health professionals to make the most of opportunities to reinforce health education.

■ Practice check

• To what extent do you consider it appropriate for limitations to be placed on a woman's choice for the sake of her fetus?

• How would you react to a mother in your care who chose a course of action that put her baby at risk?

• What support is available in your area for mothers who wish to alter their lifestyle while pregnant?

□ Acknowledgement

Thanks go to my husband, Jonathan, for his general support and encouragement, and especially for our valuable discussions on legal and ethical issues.

■ References

Aaronson LS, Macnee CL 1988 Tobacco, alcohol, and caffeine use during pregnancy. Journal of Obstetric, Gynaecologic, and Neonatal Nursing 18(4): 279–87

Barker DJP 1991 The intrauterine origins of cardiovascular and obstructive lung disease in adult life. Journal of the Royal College of Physicians of London 25(2): 129–33

Barker DJP, Osmond C, Golding J, Kuh D, Wadsworth MEJ 1989a Growth in utero, blood pressure in childhood and adult life, and mortality from cardiovascular disease. British Medical Journal 298: 564–7

Barker DJP, Winter PD, Osmond C, Margetts B, Simmonds SJ 1989b Weight in infancy and death from ischaemic heart disease. Lancet 1: 577–80

Barker DJP, Bull AR, Osmond C, Simmonds SJ 1990 Fetal and placental size and risk of hypertension in adult life. British Medical Journal 301: 259–62

Barker DJP, Gluckman PD, Godfrey KM, Harding JE, Owens JA, Robinson JS
1993 Fetal nutrition and cardiovascular disease in adult life. Lancet 341:
938–41
Committee on Substance Abuse and Committee on Children with Disabilities 1993
Fetal alcohol syndrome and fetal alcohol effects. Pediatrics 91(5): 1004–6
Eekelaar J 1988 Does a mother have legal duties to her unborn child? In Byrne P
(ed.) Health rights and resources. Oxford University Press, London, Ch 3,
p55–75
Elford J, Whincup P, Shaper AG 1991 Early life experience and adult
cardiovascular disease: longitudinal and case–control studies. International
Journal of Epidemiology 20(4): 833–44
Elford J, Shaper AG, Whincup P 1992 Early life experience and cardiovascular
disease – ecological studies. Journal of Epidemiology and Community Health
46: 1–8
Forrest F, Florey C du V, McPherson F, Young JA 1991 Reported social alcohol
consumption during pregnancy and infants' development at 18 months. British
Medical Journal 303: 22–6
Fortier I, Marcoux S, Brisson J 1994 Passive smoking during pregnancy and the risk
of delivering a small-for-gestational-age infant. American Journal of
Epidemiology 139(3): 294–301
Gillies P, Wakefield M 1993 Smoking in pregnancy. Current Obstetrics and
Gynaecology 3: 157–61
Health Education Authority 1993 Women and drinking. Health Education
Authority, London
Jones SR 1994 Ethics in midwifery. CV Mosby, Guildford
Kennedy I 1990 A woman and her unborn child: rights and responsibilities. In
Byrne P (ed.) Ethics and law in health care and research. John Wiley,
Chichester, Ch 10, p161–86
Knupfer G 1991 Abstaining for fetal health: the fiction that even light drinking is
dangerous. British Journal of Addiction 86: 1063–73
Law CM, Barker DJP, Bull AR, Osmond C 1991 Maternal and fetal influences on
blood pressure. Archives of Disease in Childhood 66: 1291–5
Lewis PJ, Boylan P 1979 Alcohol and fetal breathing. Lancet 1: 388
Long MG, Waterson EJ, MacRae KD, Murray-Lyon IM 1994 Alcohol consumption
and the risk of first trimester miscarriage. Journal of Obstetrics and
Gynaecology 14: 69–70
McLeod W, Brien J, Loomis C, Carmichael L, Probert C, Patrick J 1983 Effect of
maternal ethanol ingestion on fetal breathing movements, and heart rate at 37
to 40 weeks' gestational age. American Journal of Obstetrics and Gynecology
145(2): 251–7
Martinez FD, Wright AL, Taussig LM and the Group Health Medical Associates
1994 The effect of paternal smoking on the birthweight of newborns whose
mothers did not smoke. American Journal of Public Health 84(9): 1489–92
Mathai M, Vijayasri R, Babu S, Jeyaseelan L 1992 Passive maternal smoking and
birthweight in a South Indian population. British Journal of Obstetrics and
Gynaecology 99: 342–3
Mills JL, Graubard BI, Harley EE, Rhoads GG, Berendes HW 1984 Maternal
alcohol consumption and birth weight. Journal of the American Medical
Association 252(14): 1875–9.

Montgomery J 1994 The rights and interests of children and those with a mental handicap. In Clarke A (ed.) Genetic counselling: practice and principles. Routledge, London, Ch 9, p208–22

Newnham JP 1991 Smoking in pregnancy. Fetal Medicine Review 3: 115–32

Ogawa H, Tominaga S, Hori K, Noguchi K, Kanou I, Matsubara M 1991 Passive smoking by pregnant women and fetal growth. Journal of Epidemiology and Community Health 45: 164–8

Parazzini F, Bocciolone L, La Vecchia C, Negri E, Fedele L 1990 Maternal and paternal moderate daily alcohol consumption and unexplained miscarriages. British Journal of Obstetrics and Gynaecology 97: 618–22

Parazzini F, Tozzi L, Chatenoud L, Restelli S, Luchini L, La Vecchia C 1994 Alcohol and risk of spontaneous abortion. Human Reproduction 9(10): 1950–3

Plant M 1990 Maternal alcohol and tobacco use during pregnancy. In Alexander J, Levy V, Roch S (eds) Antenatal care: a research-based approach. Macmillan, Basingstoke, Ch 5, p73–87

Robinson RJ 1992 Introduction. In Barker DJP Fetal and infant origins of adult disease. British Medical Journal, London, p1–20

Sutherland E 1990 Regulating pregnancy: should we and can we? In Sutherland E, McCall Smith A (eds) Family rights – family law and medical advance. Edinburgh University Press, Edinburgh, Ch 6, p100–19

Taylor DJ 1993 Pregnancy alcohol consumption. Fetal and Maternal Medicine Review 5: 121–35

Thomson M 1994 After Re S. Medical Law Review 2(2): 127–48

Tolo K, Little RE 1993 Occasional binges by moderate drinkers: implications for birth outcomes. Epidemiology 4(5): 415–20

Tribe L 1979 American constitutional law. The Foundation Press, New York

Virji SK 1991 The relationship between alcohol consumption during pregnancy and infant birthweight. Acta Obstetricia et Gynaecologica Scandinavica 70: 18–21

Walpole I, Zubrick S, Pontré J, Lawrence C 1991 Low to moderate maternal alcohol use before and during pregnancy, and neurological outcome in the newborn infant. Developmental Medicine and Child Neurology 33: 875–83

Zaluska M, Bronowski P, Cendrowski K, Piotrowski A, Stelmachow J 1993 Alcohol, tobacco, and drugs during pregnancy; effect on newborn. International Journal of Prenatal and Perinatal Psychology and Medicine 5(2): 157–67

Zhang J, Ratcliffe JM 1993 Paternal smoking and birthweight in Shanghai. American Journal of Public Health 83: 207–10

■ Suggested further reading

Barker DJP 1992 Fetal and infant origins of adult disease. British Medical Journal, London

Buttriss J, Gray J 1994 Maternal and fetal nutrition. National Dairy Council, London

Jones SR 1994 Ethics in midwifery. CV Mosby, Guildford

Chapter 6

Pregnancy after treatment for infertility

Jane Denton

The rapid scientific and clinical advances in reproductive technologies have enabled many previously infertile couples to have children. It is difficult to assess the extent of infertility because of the differences in definition and lack of data (*Effective Health Care* 1992), but studies (for example Hull *et al* 1985) have suggested that as many as one in six couples may have some difficulty in conceiving. However, infertility is not a new problem, and references have been made to various ways in which it has been overcome throughout the history of the human race. One famous example is found in the Bible in the book of Genesis, where Sarah commissioned her handmaiden Hagar to bear a child for her husband Abraham, making this one of the earliest recorded cases of surrogacy.

Infertility was not widely discussed until it made international headline news in 1978 with the birth of Louise Brown, the first 'test-tube baby', which was the phrase used by the press to describe *in vitro* fertilisation (IVF). This also brought the debate about the many moral dilemmas into the public arena and the growing concern prompted the government to set up a Committee of Public Enquiry, chaired by Mary Warnock. The Warnock Report was published in 1984 (DHSS 1984) and was used as the basis for the Human Fertilisation and Embryology Act 1990 (HFE Act 1990). Prior to this, clinics offering IVF were regulated on a voluntary basis by the Interim Licensing Authority (previously the Voluntary Licensing Authority). As a result of the Act, a statutory body, the Human Fertilisation and Embryology Authority (HFEA), was established to monitor the licensing of clinics, which became a legal requirement. Any centre offering IVF, using or storing donated gametes for treatment or research, or carrying out any research involving the creation or use of human embryos must be licensed by the HFEA. A Code of Practice (HFEA 1993) provides guidance for the licensed centres. New developments continue to pose new problems, and the HFEA has to develop policies for the implementation of appropriate new techniques in clinical practice. As there is usually a wide range of views on various matters that the Authority has to consider, a public consultation is in some cases conducted. One example of this is the use of donated ovarian tissue (HFEA 1994a).

It is not the purpose of this chapter to examine the ethics of reproductive technologies in depth, but all health care workers involved with infertile couples in any capacity should have an awareness of the issues, particularly where they may have direct implications for their practice.

The definition of a successful outcome for infertility treatment is generally considered to be pregnancy, which will hopefully result in the birth of a healthy baby. However, this does not necessarily resolve the couple's complex emotional and psychological problems associated with their inability to conceive without help from external sources. As will be seen later in the chapter, having a baby can, in some cases, present a new range of anxieties, particularly when donor gametes have been used. The ways in which midwives can identify and help with these problems will be discussed.

■ It is assumed that you are already aware of the following:

- The causes of infertility;

- How infertility is diagnosed;

- The different treatments available and the indications for their use;

- The psychological and emotional consequences of being infertile.

■ The chance of pregnancy after treatment

For any individual couple, the chances of having a healthy baby will depend on many factors, including the cause of infertility and the age of the mother. It is difficult to obtain comparative data for assisted conception programmes. Different criteria are used to define the cause of infertility, and the diagnosis of early pregnancy can vary (Beral *et al* 1990). There is a need for the collection of national statistics on infertility and miscarriage (Templeton 1992). The HFEA *Annual Report* provides information about the licensed treatments. In 1992, the live birth rate per treatment cycle for IVF was 12.7 per cent and for donor insemination (DI) 5 per cent (HFEA 1994b). This clearly shows the low success rates of treatments. Studies have also indicated that the incidence of miscarriage is higher amongst infertile women, particularly those who are older. One study showed the rate of spontaneous abortion to be 15 per cent after primary infertility, 19 per cent after secondary infertility but only 7 per cent where women had conceived without difficulty (Templeton 1992). The risk of ectopic pregnancy after IVF has been shown to be between 2 and 11 per cent, which is higher than after spontaneous conception (Marcus and Brinsden (1995)). The incidence of multiple pregnancy after assisted conception procedures is much higher than with spontaneous conception (MRC Working Party 1990; Ghazi *et al* 1991). The number of triplets and higher order births in the UK has increased threefold since the mid 1980s. In 1983, 7233 twins and 95 sets of triplets were delivered, compared with 9362 sets of twins and 253 sets of triplets in 1993. A national survey in 1989 showed that two-thirds of triplets resulted from infertility treatment (Levene *et al* 1992). The HFEA *Annual report* of 1994 indicated that, after IVF, the incidence of multiple pregnancy was 29 per cent, whereas it is about 1 per cent after spontaneous conceptions (HFEA 1994b).

Although there is a great deal of information about the scientific and clinical aspects of infertility treatment, especially IVF and associated techniques, most studies so far have looked only at the reproductive outcomes. Ideally, the effectiveness of infertility treatments should also be evaluated in relation to the resolution of social and psychological difficulties (*Effective Health Care* 1992). Follow-up studies, ideally on an international basis, are also needed to provide large series of data, particularly to assess the outcome for babies born as a result of new techniques such as intracytoplasmic sperm injection (ICSI).

☐ **Diagnosis of pregnancy**

The diagnosis of pregnancy is usually made much earlier than after a spontaneous conception. Because the cycle is so carefully monitored, the exact time of ovulation is usually known, and a pregnancy test can be performed as soon as a period is a day or two late. In many infertility clinics, patients also have an early ultrasound scan at between 6 and 8 weeks gestation. There are two main reasons for this. First, there is an increased risk of multiple pregnancy if three embryos have been replaced or if there has been multiple ovulation. An early diagnosis of an ectopic pregnancy can also be made and appropriate treatment given. Second, the HFEA (1993) has a legal obligation to maintain a register of the outcome of all treatment cycles resulting from IVF or DI, and the HFEA defines a clinical pregnancy as the presence of a fetal heart on ultrasound scan. This information must be submitted to the HFEA.

Many people assume that as soon as a pregnancy is diagnosed, the couple will be overjoyed. Although there may be initial joy, this is often quickly followed by intense anxiety about the pregnancy and the risk of loss. Couples may have spent many years trying to come to terms with their infertility and part of their coping mechanisms for repeated failure of treatment may have been to refuse to think about actually being pregnant (Bernstein 1990). Most specialist infertility clinics do not offer obstetric services, so it is likely that the couple will be advised to book in for routine antenatal care near to their home. If the doctor and midwife are unaware of the previous infertility, they may fail to appreciate the stress and need for support and reassurance that the pregnancy is going well (Sandelowski *et al* 1990). It can be quite disconcerting to find that after possibly years of treatment, with intensive care and interest in every day of the treatment cycle, a woman finds that she is now regarded as 'ordinary' and told that there is no need to book in for antenatal care for several weeks yet. Alternatively some women, fearing that the pregnancy will not continue, may not seek help for many weeks (Garner 1985).

■ Early pregnancy loss

An early scan may well reveal more than one gestation sac or fetal heart. It has now been established that the chance of one or more of the fetuses failing to survive is high. This is known as the vanishing twin syndrome (Landy *et al* 1982; Goldman *et al* 1989) and also occurs in spontaneous pregnancies, although it would not usually be recognised as scans would rarely be carried out at this early stage. There is wide debate about the status of an embryo and about when exactly human life begins (Dunstan 1990). Many would not consider that an embryo that implanted but failed to thrive had the same importance as a baby dying in later pregnancy. However, to many couples, particularly after IVF when each embryo has been individually identified and carefully replaced, they may all be regarded as precious babies (Sandelowski *et al* 1990). The strength of the mother's feelings has been shown to be increased once the fetuses have been seen on ultrasound scan (Campbell *et al* 1992), and the sense of loss and grieving should not be underestimated.

Garner (1985) points out that women who have had previous ectopic pregnancies or spontaneous abortions after infertility treatment need particular understanding from the midwife. To them, their infertility is not just the problem of conceiving but also the inability of their body to carry a pregnancy. They see themselves as failures and are fearful of another pregnancy and a possible repeat of the loss.

Should fetal loss occur, the next question that the couple will have to consider is whether and when to start trying again to conceive. After a spontaneous conception, it is usual to suggest waiting until the menstrual cycle is established again and also to allow time for the grieving process. However, the infertile couple faces a different situation as the woman is likely to be older (Bowman & Saunders 1995; Lansac 1995) and to need assistance again. An appointment should be made to review the situation with the infertility specialist as soon as the couple wish it. Counselling should be offered at the same time.

■ Antenatal care

Infertile couples may choose not to reveal that they have had help to achieve the pregnancy, and midwives should be aware of this. Disproportionate anxiety and stress may alert the midwife, but she must respect the couple's decision, which should be borne in mind when record keeping. Maintaining confidentiality is a factor that is addressed in the HFE Act and HFEA Code of Practice (1993), and it is a criminal offence for anybody working in a centre licensed by the HFEA to pass on information relating to licensed treatments without the patient's consent (HFE Act 1990). This demonstrates the concern over the sensitivity of this information, and it is important that midwives are aware of this. Some couples may specifically request that certain details about the conception, for example the use of donor sperm, are not written anywhere in the records. (The use of donor sperm is discussed below.)

If the couple are open about the method of conception, sensitive questioning may encourage discussion, and it may be a relief for the mother to acknowledge some of her fears and concerns and accept support from the midwife. As Garner (1985) suggests, the midwife has a significant role to play with infertile couples, and this is an ideal time to educate and reassure them. Continuity of care is essential to build up a trusting relationship in such a situation.

The question of prenatal screening may present the couple with a painful dilemma. Mothers who have conceived after infertility treatment are likely to be older (Lansac 1995) and therefore more likely to be offered routine screening, usually initially blood tests, depending of course on the local policy.

Consideration must be given not only to the risk of miscarriage after procedures such as amniocentesis, but also to the course of action that would be taken should the results indicate that the baby (or one of the babies in a multiple pregnancy) had abnormalities. An older mother who has had many years of infertility treatment and might not easily achieve another pregnancy may wish to decline the tests. Careful counselling should be available to these couples and appropriate support provided, whatever their decision.

With a multiple pregnancy, a scan should be performed in the first trimester to establish chorionicity (Fisk & Bryan 1993). Many professionals as well as parents assume that if there was multiple follicular development after induction of ovulation, or up to three embryos were replaced after IVF, the babies must be dizygotic, but this is not always the case. It appears that embryo division may be more common after ovulation induction and IVF than after spontaneous conception (Derom *et al* 1987; Wenstrom *et al* 1993). More data are required about this as it may have implications for the number of embryos that are replaced per cycle.

Anxiety during pregnancy is generally to be expected (Reading *et al* 1989). However, a small study by Stanton and Golombok (1993) of 15 women who had conceived after IVF and had reached at least 20 weeks gestation, compared with a control group of 20 women with spontaneous conceptions, showed that mothers who had conceived after IVF did not have higher anxiety levels than those who had conceived spontaneously. They concluded that the anxiety shown during IVF treatment was diminished once pregnancy was achieved. However, the same group were more negative about their marital and social relationships, which may have been associated with their infertility. Larger studies are required to assess anxiety and attitudes towards the pregnancy in order to identify ways in which midwives may need to adapt their care to meet the needs of these mothers.

■ **Method of delivery**

There is little information available about delivery after infertility treatment. However, higher rates of caesarean section are reported (Varma *et al* 1988; Ghazi *et al* 1991; Tan *et al* 1992). One of the largest studies (Venn & Lumley 1993) found that the caesarean section rate was more than doubled in the group of women who had a history of infertility. As expected after induction of ovulation, IVF and gamete intrafallopian transfer (GIFT) procedures, multiple pregnancies were more common in the infertility group, which was one of the reasons for the increase in the rate of caesarean section. However, overall, the indications for caesarean section were significantly different between the infertility and control groups, and it seemed that less severe complications led to caesarean section being performed in the former. It has been suggested that anxiety on the part of the obstetricians and parents is a reason for the increased rate (Li *et al* 1991; Tan *et al* 1992).

■ **Outcome of pregnancies after infertility treatment**

This is another area in which more data are required. There are inevitably concerns about the possible damage that might occur to the gametes and embryos when they are subjected to new techniques and fertilisation takes place outside the body. ICSI, which involves injecting a single sperm into the cytoplasm of the oocyte, is proving to be a major advance in treatment when the male partner has a very low sperm count (Van Steirteghem *et al* 1993). Although the results to date do not indicate a high risk of abnormality, long-term follow-up studies are essential (*Effective Health Care* 1992).

The Medical Research Council Working Party (1990) compared the characteristics at birth of children in the UK conceived after IVF and GIFT between 1978 and 1987 with the national statistics. It was shown that 24 per cent of these births were preterm, as opposed to 6 per cent after spontaneous conception. Rates of stillbirth and neonatal and infant death were about twice the national average. Thirty-two per cent of the babies weighed less than 2500 g, compared with 7 per cent for all births in England and Wales for the same period, with 7 per cent weighing less than 1500 g, compared with 1 per cent in England and Wales. The reason for these differences is almost entirely explained by the high number of multiple births. The incidence of congenital malformations was no higher than in the general population, which was also confirmed in a study by Rizk *et al* (1991). Similar trends have been reported from studies in other countries with ongoing IVF programmes (Lancaster 1985; Ghazi *et al* 1991; Rufat *et al* 1994). More research is needed to follow up children in the longer term to assess the risk of problems when they are older (*Effective Health Care* 1992).

■ Multiple births

'Nobody goes to a fertility clinic and says "Doctor, I'd love to have triplets" – you just put up with it', commented one mother (Bryan pers comm 1989). The dramatic increase in the number of multiple births after infertility treatment is well documented (Botting 1992). Although many would regard having more than one child to be an ideal outcome after many years of infertility treatment, this is often far from the case.

The anecdotal reports in the late 1980s of the problems of multiple birth families and the increasing pressure on neonatal intensive care services prompted a national study of triplet and higher order births. This was undertaken collaboratively between the Office of Population Censuses and Surveys, the Child Care and Development Group of the University of Cambridge and the National Perinatal Epidemiology Unit. *Three, Four and More: A Study of Triplet and Higher Order Births* (the National Triplet Study) was published in 1990 (Botting *et al* 1990) and is essential reading for any professionals involved with multiple birth families. The major factors that emerged were the lack of under-standing and knowledge of professionals about the concerns and needs of the parents, and the practical and financial problems that the families faced.

Spillman (1990) reviewed the anxieties of multiple birth parents and the implications for midwifery practice. There are additional points that midwives should take into account when multiple birth results from treatment for infertility.

The HFEA has limited the number of embryos that can be replaced after IVF to a maximum of three, which has helped to reduce the risk of high order multiple pregnancies, but in 1992 (HFEA 1994b) 24 per cent of pregnancies after IVF were twin and 4 per cent triplet. The overall multiple birth rate following IVF was 31.3 per cent. The policy in some infertility units is now changing to replacing only two embryos, to reduce the risk of multiple pregnancy for women who are more likely to conceive, such as a woman under 30 years of age who has tubal damage. The HFEA Code of Practice requires all patients having treatment in licensed centres to be given information about the 'possible side effects and risks of the treatment to the woman and resulting child, including where relevant the risks associated with multiple pregnancy' (HFEA 1993: 21). However, although this is good practice, the same amount of information and offer of counselling is not always given to those couples having non-licensed treatments. Many consider that ovulation induction with gonadotrophic hormone preparations should also be subject to more rigorous control (Levene *et al* 1992). The Royal College of Obstetricians and Gynaecologists (1994) has published guidelines recommending that 'in general regimens which minimise or avoid the risk of multiple pregnancy even at the expense of lower pregnancy rates' should be used. A prospective study of triplets and higher order births in 1989 by Levene *et al* (1992) revealed that 34 per cent were conceived after ovarian stimulation using clomiphene or gonadotrophins, 24 per cent after IVF and 11 per cent after GIFT. Another controversial aspect of the rising numbers of multiple births highlighted in this study is the increased demand on neonatal intensive care facilities as a result of the preterm births (see below).

Seventy-one per cent of the women in the National Triplet Study reported that there had been some discussion about multiple birth, but some had been given reassuring advice, 1 per cent were told that the treatment would be controlled and 4 per cent were led to believe that even twins were unlikely (Botting *et al* 1990). One woman who conceived triplets after clomiphene citrate was prescribed for anovulation commented: 'My consultant simply said that there was no risk of a multiple pregnancy' (Botting *et al* 1990: 55).

A survey by Linney (1994) to assess mental health promotion needs of 48 mothers who had multiple births after infertility treatment showed that they would have liked more information and counselling on the chances of having a multiple pregnancy and the risks and consequences of preterm birth.

In the National Triplet Study (Botting *et al* 1990), half the women who had infertility treatment had their triplets (or more) diagnosed by ultrasound scan before 12 weeks gestation, but this happened in only 13 per cent of cases after spontaneous conception.

Linney (1994) found that the reaction to the news varied from shock and disbelief to pleasure and surprise. Forty-four out of the 48 said that they were given no counselling at this stage, and 19 said, surprisingly, that they had no named professional looking after them.

The anxiety experienced by couples after infertility treatment is likely to be increased by a multiple pregnancy. There are not only the additional risks to the pregnancy with a higher chance of spontaneous abortion and obstetric complications, such as pre-eclampsia and poly-hydramnios (MacGillivray 1991), but also an increased chance of preterm delivery, with its associated neonatal complications (Cooke 1991). The couple may also feel overwhelmed by the thought of caring for two or more babies, and their immediate concerns are often related to the practical and financial aspects of caring for their families. The potential emotional difficulties should not be underestimated, as parents may wonder whether they will be able to relate to each child equally and give each the same opportunities they envisaged for the one baby they had expected if the infertility treatment were successful.

As much information as possible should be provided, and Linney (1994) found that contact with other parents with similar experiences and with support groups was very valuable. The Multiple Births Founda-tion (MBF) offers support to families as soon as a multiple pregnancy is diagnosed. It provides advice to couples on an individual basis and also to groups through prenatal meetings. Support is offered to families with twins or more of all ages through specialist clinics and telephone consul-tations. Local Twin Clubs, which can be contacted through the umbrella organisation the Twins and Multiple Births Association (TAMBA), are an excellent source of information. TAMBA also has an Infertility Support Group for those who have multiple births as a result of treatment.

■ Antenatal and postnatal care

The preparation for delivery should ideally include a special parentcraft class for those expecting a multiple birth. The MBF (Davies 1995) has developed an education pack to assist midwives and health visitors in establishing local classes based on the MBF Prenatal Meetings, which are held every 2 months in London.

One of the major concerns of the parents will be how they will cope with all these babies. It is often wrongly assumed that if they have paid for private infertility treatment, they will be able to afford to pay for help. When undertaking treatment, most couples assume success to mean that one baby will be born and that the mother will be able to return to work should she wish. However, if twins or more are the result, it may not be financially viable to do this as the cost of childcare can be greater than the second income (Botting *et al* 1990). Unplanned expenditure is almost inevitable as the family will require extra equipment for two or more babies, to say nothing of the possible need for a larger house or car.

There is no statutory requirement for the provision of either practical or financial support. Although the social services are able to offer limited assistance in some cases, this is increasingly difficult to obtain with the demand for limited resources. It is helpful if the midwife can liaise with the health visitor antenatally so that postnatal care and support can be organised well ahead, giving some reassurance to the mother.

It will help to allay some of the anxieties if the parents are consulted and fully informed about the plan for the management of the pregnancy and delivery. The National Triplet Study (Botting *et al* 1990) found that there was a higher caesarean section rate for triplets and higher order births conceived after infertility treatment, which was suggested to be due to the concern of the parents and obstetricians to deliver the babies 'successfully'.

A visit to the neonatal unit should be arranged early in the pregnancy, bearing in mind that the delivery is likely to be preterm (Spillman 1990).

The increase in multiple births from treatment for infertility has brought additional pressures on neonatal intensive care units. As reported in the National Triplet Study (Botting *et al* 1990), mothers may need to be transferred to other hospitals if intensive care cots are not available when a preterm delivery is imminent. Close collaboration between the midwife, obstetrician and paediatricians, and careful planning, should help to reduce the chance of this, but in some cases it is unavoidable. It is preferable to keep the mother and babies together, although there continue to be situations in which the mother may be in one hospital with one or more of the babies in another. This, of course, puts an enormous strain on the parents, who are already distressed about their sick infants.

Midwives should also be aware of the increased risk of postnatal depression as the result of a multiple birth after infertility treatment. Thorpe *et al* (1991) found a higher incidence of depression in mothers of twins, and other studies (Hay *et al* 1990; Spillman 1992) have shown increased exhaustion and anxiety in mothers of multiple babies, linked to the depression. Bernstein *et al* (1985) suggest that the mother who had feelings of inadequacy associated with her infertility may be at high risk of postnatal depression. Thorough prenatal preparation and good postnatal support should help to avoid this.

■ Bereavement

Higher perinatal mortality rates with multiple births continue despite improvements in obstetric and neonatal care. Botting *et al* (1987) found that in the UK, twins account for about 2 per cent of births but 9 per cent of perinatal deaths.

The needs of the parents and the surviving child or children have been well documented by Elizabeth Bryan (1992). The grief accompanying the complete loss of a multiple pregnancy after infertility treatment is likely to be acknowledged. However, when there is a survivor, the parents' grief is often underestimated, and they are forced to suppress their grief for the babies who have died, each of whom is equally important and valued (Bryan 1991). Midwives and other professionals involved should be aware of this and support the parents appropriately.

■ Embryo reduction

Embryo reduction is an option that some couples may consider when a triplet or higher order pregnancy is confirmed.

This procedure may be carried out if the requirements of the 1967 Abortion Act, as amended by section 17 of the 1990 HFE Act, are met. Most couples, and indeed many professionals, have never heard of the procedure. Couples are often deeply shocked to find out that it can be done, and they are then faced with an immensely difficult decision, although some people of course know that they could not consent to any of their babies being destroyed. The information and counselling on the implications and possible consequences of infertility treatment that is offered to patients before starting treatment often does not cover this subject. It is difficult to raise the subject of embryo reduction at a time when everything is focused on producing a pregnancy, but couples who have contacted the Multiple Births Foundation frequently feel angry that they were not informed before starting treatment that they may be confronted with this dilemma (personal experience).

Parents considering a reduction have to face the risk of miscarriage, the possible harm to the other babies, and the emotional and psychological aspects of coping with the procedure, compared with the higher risk of premature birth, with its associated mortality and morbidity, and the practical financial and emotional factors associated with having triplets or more. The couple may choose not to tell any of the staff involved with their care that they have had an embryo reduction, or they may choose to tell just their midwife and ask for this not to be discussed with other members of the team. Sensitive support from the midwife and awareness of the potential emotional difficulties, particularly at delivery, when the parents will inevitably think of the other baby or babies who might also have been born, will be invaluable in helping these parents to come to terms with the situation.

■ Selective fetocide

Couples may also face a difficult decision if one baby is found to have major abnormalities, and selective fetocide has to be considered. Bryan (1989) describes the importance of identifying and clarifying the emotional issues raised, and the midwife will play a crucial role in helping the parents to acknowledge the bereavement and to grieve for the dead baby.

More research into the emotional and psychological outcomes of embryo reduction and selective fetocide is required to enable carers fully to support these couples, not only throughout the pregnancy and delivery, but also in the longer term. The MBF have information leaflets for couples about both procedures.

■ Donor gametes

Although donor sperm have been used for many years to overcome infertility, it is only with IVF procedures that is has been possible to use donor eggs. There are many complex ethical, emotional and psychological issues around the use of donated gametes, but for the purposes of this chapter, it is the role of the midwife that will be specifically considered.

Although some studies on outcome of DI are available (Amuzu *et al* 1990; Snowden 1990; Oskarson *et al* 1991; Golombok *et al* 1995), more information is needed about the longer-term outcomes. There is very little about the use of donated eggs and the outcome of the pregnancies, although some studies are underway. One of the difficulties with follow-up is the sensitivity and privacy that surround the treatment, and, as Amuzu found in her study (1990), this will constrain the information that becomes available. The question of whether to tell anybody at all about the use of donated gametes provokes much debate. Snowden (1990) voices the concern of many about the possible consequences of keeping a secret and risking the child finding out accidentally about his or her genetic origins, which could result in great distress for all concerned. The HFEA Code of Practice (1993) requires licensed centres to offer counselling on the implications of the treatment, including inviting couples to consider 'the advantages and disadvantages of openness about the procedures envisaged and how they might be explained to relatives and friends; their feelings about not being the genetic parents of the child; their perceptions of the needs of the child throughout his or her childhood and adolescence' (HFEA 1993: 30). Amuzu's study (1990) of 427 women who conceived after DI showed that the majority of couples (71.7 per cent) told their obstetricians about the method of conception, but half did not tell their family or friends. When asked about telling the children, 47 per cent said they definitely would not, 14 per cent thought they probably would not, 13 per cent said they would, 5 per cent said that they probably would, while 21 per cent remained un-decided. Golombok *et al* (1995) found that none of the parents in their study had told their children, but suggested that the study involved couples who had received treatment prior to the HFE Act 1990 who had not therefore necessarily had the same opportunity for the counselling specified in the HFEA Code of Practice (HFEA 1993); future studies may therefore differ. Anecdotal feedback at present still suggests that many couples at the time of treatment and conception feel that they will not tell the child of its genetic origins.

The implications for the midwife are complex. She must be aware of and respect the couple's wishes and offer appropriate support. There may be additional anxiety at the delivery. Although DI treatments are rigorously controlled, the couple may be anxious that the baby will be of a different ethnic group or look completely unlike either of them. They may also have concerns about how they will relate to this baby. Information about the position relating to the legal fatherhood of the baby will have been given to the couple by the infertility clinic. The husband or partner of the woman is regarded as the legal father unless he specifically did not consent to the treatment (HMSO 1990). If the midwife considered that further counselling might be helpful after the birth, it would be advisable for the couple to contact the clinic where they received their treatment. Alternatively, the British Infertility Counselling Association may be able to help (see 'Useful addresses' below).

The information that should be made available to children conceived as a result of using donated gametes is also a much debated matter (Morgan & Lee 1991). One of the concerns is the risk of consanguinity that could arise if a man and woman born from the same donor married or had a child. The HFE Act 1990 now requires the HFEA to keep a register of all treatments using donated gametes, and it is essential that parents tell infertility clinics the birth details to enable them to fulfil their legal obligation of informing the HFEA. Although no identifying information about the donor will be given, anybody reaching the age of 18 (or 16 if they are planning to marry) can ask the HFEA if they were born as a result of gamete donation and if they are related to their proposed partner.

Donors known to the couple may be used, but the general guidance in circumstances laid down in the HFEA Code of Practice (1993) must be followed. This is a practice that is open to debate, many people believing that donation should be anonymous (Templeton 1991). This probably happens more often with donated eggs when sisters or friends provide the gametes. Midwives should consider and be aware of the complex emotions that are likely to surround the birth.

There is a shortage of egg donors, and it is likely that the demands will continue to increase (Templeton 1991). Midwives may well find themselves asked about how to donate, and the best advice would probably be to refer the woman to the National Egg and Embryo Donation Society (NEEDS; see 'Useful addresses' below).

■ Surrogacy

Commercial surrogacy in the UK is banned by the Surrogacy Arrangements Act 1985, but it is allowed on a non-commercial basis and is increasingly being offered through infertility clinics. The HFEA Code of Practice stipulates that 'a surrogate pregnancy should only be considered where it is physically impossible or highly undesirable for medical reasons for the commissioning mother to carry the child' (HFEA 1993: 15). Infertility clinics are required to offer appropriate counselling for the commissioning parents and host mother. It is desirable that the midwife is involved in the plans as soon as possible after the pregnancy has been confirmed, as she will have to take into account not only the host mother who is carrying the baby, but also the commissioning parents who will be caring for the child from birth and who will probably be very anxious and eager to know all the details of the ongoing pregnancy. The delivery and support for all concerned should be well planned and the obstetric team fully informed of the arrangements.

The surrogate parents, that is, the birth mother and her husband or partner, are legally the parents of the child until legal parentage is transferred to the commissioning couple. Regulations, implementing Section 30 of the Human Fertilisation and Embryology Act (1990) which came into effect on 1 November 1994, introduce parental orders which allow parental rights and obligations to be transferred to the commissioning parents, thus speeding up the process that would in the past have been through an adoption procedure. The commissioning couple must have applied for an order within 6 months of the child's birth, and one of them must be genetically related to the child. The couple must also be married. Midwives should be aware of these procedures. Further advice can be obtained from the Department of Health.

■ Future developments

The use of ovarian tissue from either dead women or aborted fetuses could in the future be a source of eggs used to create embryos for use by infertile women or for research. This has already provoked great interest, and the HFEA conducted a public consultation on the subject. The report was published in 1994 (HFEA 1994c). It concluded that if further research proves that ovarian tissue is a viable source of oocytes, the HFEA would allow in treatment the use of such tissue from live women but not from cadavers or fetuses. The use of tissue from all three sources was considered to be acceptable for research, but only subject to existing controls.

Issues such as this, the use of preimplantation diagnosis and sex selection, which are already much debated (Marteau 1993; Hook 1994), will continue to arise with scientific advances, and midwives should seek to keep abreast of developments to help to anticipate the future needs of their clients.

■ Conclusions

The major advances in infertility treatment have not yet been sufficiently followed up to allow evaluation of the outcomes. Comprehensive collaborative international studies are required to enable us to assess fully not only the clinical and scientific results, but also the psychological and emotional impact of these treatments on the parents and resulting children.

The information available suggests that there are no major detrimental outcomes. However, even with good follow-up studies, it will be many years before some aspects, such as the potential carcinogenic effects of the ovulation-stimulating drugs on the ovary (Whittemore 1994) and the long-term effects of freezing embryos, can be analysed. The psychological and social elements will only be fully revealed when the children reach adulthood (Bryan & Higgins 1995).

In the meantime, practice must reflect the knowledge we have, combined with high standards of professional care, support and sensitivity for the potentially difficult situations that these couples face.

■ Recommendations for clinical practice in the light of currently available evidence

1. Midwives should be aware of the different types of infertility treatment available and the legal framework that controls the treatments licensed by the HFEA.

2. Pre- and postregistration programmes for midwives should include relevant information. Frequent review is necessary to ensure that the

latest techniques are included and potential and future ethical issues considered.

3. Close liaison with infertility centres would ensure continuity of care, but confidentiality and the couple's wishes must be established and respected.

4. Midwives should be aware of the complex emotional factors surrounding a pregnancy after infertility treatment, provide as much information and reassurance as possible and acknowledge the additional anxieties.

5. Midwives should instigate and participate in research in this area as opportunities arise.

■ Practice check

- Do you always consider whether a pregnancy may be the result of treatment for infertility?

- Do you have any formal contact with local infertility clinics? If not, would this be helpful for the staff and for couples who conceive after treatment?

- How do you broach the subject of whether conception was a result of treatment, and what action would you take if the mother's reply differed from the information in the doctor's referral letter?

    How would you ensure that confidentiality was maintained, taking into account the couple's wishes and the need for your colleagues to be fully aware of the implications of information relevant to the case?

    Would the management plan differ if the conception were a result of IVF?

- What additional information and support is available for women with a multiple pregnancy?

- How would you support a woman who had a selective fetocide in a twin pregnancy that was ongoing after the procedure?

- Are you aware of the bereavement policies and procedures in your unit?

- Reflect on your personal views relating to the ethics of the treatments and procedures discussed in this chapter. How might your views influence the care you give?

■ References

Amuzu B, Laxova R, Shapiro SS 1990 Pregnancy outcome, health of children, and family adjustment after donor insemination. Obstetrics and Gynecology 75(6): 899–905

Beral V, Doyle P, Tan SL, Mason BA, Campbell S 1990 Outcome of pregnancies resulting from assisted conception. In Edwards RG (ed.) Assisted human conception   46(3): 753–68

Bernstein J 1990 Parenting after infertility. Journal of Perinatal and Neonatal Nursing   4(2): 11–23

Bernstein J, Potts N, Mattox J 1985 Assessment of psychological dysfunction associated with infertility. JOGNN   14(6): s63–6

Botting BJ, Macdonald Davies I, Macfarlane A 1987 Recent trends in the incidence of multiple births and associated mortality. Archives of Disease in Childhood 62: 941–50

Botting BJ, Macfarlane FJ, Price FV 1990 Three, four and more: a study of triplet and higher order births. HMSO, London

Botting BJ 1992 Reproductive trends in the UK. In Templeton AA, Drife JO (eds) Infertility. Springer–Verlag, Berlin, Ch 1, p3–22

Bowman M, Saunders DM 1995 Are the risks of delayed parenting overstated? Human Reproduction   10(5): 1035–6

Bryan E 1989 The response of mothers to selective feticide. Ethical Problems in Reproductive Medicine   1: 28–30

Bryan E 1991 But there should have been two. In Harvey D, Bryan E (eds) The stress of multiple births. The Multiple Births Foundation, London, Ch 5, p49–58

Bryan E 1992 Twins and higher multiple births. A guide to their nature and nurture. Edward Arnold, London

Bryan E, Higgins R 1995 Priorities for research. In Infertility: new choices, new dilemmas. Penguin, Harmondsworth, Ch 16, p224–30

Campbell S, Reading AE, Cox DN 1982 Ultrasound scanning in pregnancy: the short term psychological effects of early real time scans. Journal of Psychosomatic Obstetrics and Gynaecology   1: 57–61

Cooke R 1991 Neonatal problems. In Harvey D, Bryan E (eds) The stress of multiple births. Multiple Births Foundation, London, Ch 4, p43–8

Davies M 1995 Educating parents for multiple births. Modern Midwife   5(11): 10–14

Department of Health and Social Security 1984 Report of the Committee of Inquiry into Human Fertilisation and Embryology (the Warnock Report). HMSO, London

Derom C, Derom R, Vlietinck R, Van Den Berghe H, Thiery M 1987 Increased monozygotic twinning rate after ovulation induction. Lancet   May 30: 1236–8

Dunstan G 1990 The moral status of the human embryo. In Bromham R, Dalton ME, Jackson JC (eds) Philosophical ethics in reproductive medicine. Manchester University Press, Manchester, Ch 1, p3–14

Effective Health Care 1992 The management of subfertility. *Effective Health Care* No 3. School of Public Health, University of Leeds

Fisk NM, Bryan EM 1993 Routine prenatal determination of chorionicity in multiple gestation – a plea to the obstetrician. British Journal of Obstetrics and Gynaecology   100: 975–7

Garner CH 1985 Pregnancy after infertility. JOGNN   November/December: s58–62

Ghazi HA, Spielberger C, Kallen B 1991 Delivery outcome after infertility – a registry study. Fertility and Sterility   55(4): 726–32

Goldman GA, Dicker D, Feldberg D, Ashkenazi J, Yeshaya A, Goldman JA 1989 The vanishing fetus. A report of 17 cases of triplets and quadruplets. Journal of Perinatal Medicine   17: 157–61

Golombok S, Cook R, Bish A, Murray C 1995 Families created by the new reproductive technologies: quality of parenting and social and emotional development of the children. Child Development   66: 285–98

Hay DA, Gleeson C, Davies C, Lordon B, Mitchell D, Paton L 1990 What information should the multiple birth family receive before, during and after the birth? Acta Geneticae Medicae Gemellologiae/Twin Research 39: 259–69

Hull MGR, Glazener CMA, Kelly NJ, Conway DI, Foster PA, Hinton RA, Coulson C, Lambert PA, Watt EM, Desai KM 1985 Population study of causes, treatment and outcome of infertility. British Medical Journal 291: 1693–7

Human Fertilisation and Embryology Act 1990. HMSO, London

Human Fertilisation and Embryology Authority 1993 Code of practice. HFEA, London

Human Fertilisation and Embryology Authority 1994a Donated ovarian tissue in embryo research and assisted conception. Public Consultation Document. HFEA, London

Human Fertilisation and Embryology Authority 1994b Third annual report. HFEA, London

Human Fertilisation and Embryology Authority 1994c Donated ovarian tissue in embryo research and assisted conception. HFEA, London

Hook EB 1994 Prenatal sex selection and autonomous reproductive decision. British Medical Journal   343: 55–6

Lancaster PAL 1985 High incidence of preterm births and early losses in pregnancy after in vitro fertilisation. British Medical Journal   291: 1160–3

Landy HJ, Keith L, Keith D 1982 The vanishing twin. Acta Geneticae Medicae Gemellologiae/Twin Research   31(3/4): 179–94

Lansac J 1995 Delayed parenting. Is delayed childbearing a good thing? Human Reproduction   10(5): 1033–5

Levene MI, Wild J, Steer P 1992 Higher multiple births and the modern management of infertility in Britain. British Journal of Obstetrics and Gynaecology   99: 607–13

Li TC, Macleod I, Singal V, Duncan SLB 1991 The obstetric and neonatal outcome of pregnancy in women with a previous history of infertility: a prospective study. British Journal of Obstetrics and Gynaecology   98: 1087–92

Linney J 1994 Multiple births: assessing the health promotion needs of mothers who have had multiple births as a result of infertility. Unpublished dissertation submitted in partial fulfilment of the degree of MSc in Health Education and Promotion, South Bank University, London

MacGillivray I 1991 Obstetrical aspects of multiple births. In Harvey D, Bryan E (eds) The stress of multiple births. Multiple Births Foundation, London, Ch 1, p11–21

Marcus SF, Brinsden PR 1995 Analysis of the incidence and risk factors associated with ectopic pregnancy following in-vitro fertilization and embryo transfer. Human Reproduction 10(1): 199–203

Marteau TM 1993 Sex selection: 'the rights of man' or the thin edge of the wedge? British Medical Journal 306: 1704–5

Medical Research Council Working Party on Children Conceived by In Vitro Fertilisation 1990 Births in Great Britain resulting from assisted conception, 1978–87. British Medical Journal 300: 1229–33

Morgan D, Lee RG 1991 Human Fertilisation and Embryology Act 1990 Abortion and embryo research, the new law. Blackstone Press, London

Oskarsson T, Dimitry ES, Mills MS, Hunt J, Winston RML 1991 Attitudes towards gamete donation among couples undergoing in vitro fertilisation. British Journal of Obstetrics and Gynaecology 98: 351–6

Reading AE, Chang LC, Kerin J 1989 Attitudes and anxiety levels in women conceiving through in vitro fertilization and gamete intrafallopian transfer. Fertility and Sterility 52(1): 95–9

Rizk B, Doyle P, Tan SL, Rainsbury P, Betts J, Brihsden P, Edwards R 1991 Perinatal outcome and congenital malformations in in-vitro fertilization babies from the Bourn Hallam Group. Human Reproduction 6(9): 1259–64

Royal College of Obstetricians and Gynaecologists 1994 RCOG guidelines: use of gonadotrophic hormone preparations for ovulation induction. RCOG, London

Rufat P, Olivennes F, Mouzon J, Dehan M, Frydman R 1994 Task force report on the outcome of pregnancies and children conceived by in vitro fertilisation (France 1987 to 1989). Fertility and Sterility 61(2): 324–30

Sandelowski M, Harris BG, Holditch-Davis D 1990 Pregnant moments: the process of conception in infertile couples. Research in Nursing and Health 13: 273–82

Snowden R 1990 The family and artificial reproduction. In Bromham DR, Dalton ME, Jackson JC (eds) Philosophical ethics in reproductive medicine. Manchester University Press, Manchester, Ch 2, p70–83

Spillman J 1990 Multiple births – parents' anxieties and the realities. In Alexander J, Levy V, Roch S (eds) Antenatal care: a research-based approach. Macmillan, Basingstoke, Ch 9, p134–48

Spillman JR 1992 A study of maternal provision in the UK in response to the needs of families who have a multiple birth. Acta Geneticae Medicae Gemellologiae/Twin Research 41: 353–64

Stanton F, Golombok S 1993 Maternal–fetal attachment during pregnancy following in vitro fertilization. Journal of Psychosomatic Obstetrics and Gynaecology 14: 153–8

Surrogacy Arrangements Act 1985. HMSO, London

Tan SL, Doyle P, Campbell S, Beral V, Rizk B, Brinsden P, Mason B, Edwards RG 1992 Obstetric outcome of in vitro fertilization pregnancies compared with normally conceived pregnancies. American Journal of Obstetrics and Gynecology 167: 778–84

Templeton A 1991 Gamete donation and anonymity. British Journal of Obstetrics and Gynaecology 98: 343–50

Templeton A 1992 The epidemiology of infertility. In Templeton AA, Drife JO (eds) Infertility. Springer-Verlag, Berlin, Ch 2, p23–32

Thorpe K, Golding J, MacGillivray I, Greenwood R 1991 Comparison of depression in mothers of twins and mothers of singletons. British Medical Journal 302: 875–8

Van Steirteghem AC, Nagy Z, Joris H, Liu J, Staessen C, Smitz J, Wisanto A, Devroey P 1993 High fertilization and implantation rates after intracytoplasmic sperm injection. Human Reproduction 8(7): 1061–6

Varma TR, Patel RH, Bhathenia RK 1988 Outcome of pregnancy after infertility. Acta Obstetricia et Gynecologica Scandinavica 67: 115–19

Venn A, Lumley J 1993 Births after a period of infertility in Victorian women 1982–1990. Australia and New Zealand Journal of Obstetrics and Gynaecology 33(4): 379–84

Wenstrom KD, Syrop CH, Hammit DG, VanVoorhis BJ 1993 Increased risk of monochorionic twinning associated with assisted reproduction. Fertility and Sterility 60(3): 510–14

Whittemore A 1994 The risk of ovarian cancer after treatment for infertility. New England Journal of Medicine 331(12): 805–6

■ Suggested further reading

Botting BJ, Macfarlane AJ, Price FV 1991 Three, four and more: a study of triplet and higher order births. HMSO, London

Bryan E, Higgins R 1995 Infertility: new choices, new dilemmas. Penguin, Harmondsworth

Jennings SE 1995 Infertility counselling. Blackwell Scientific, London

Meerabeau L, Denton J 1995 Infertility: nursing and caring. Scutari Press, London

Morgan D, Lee RG 1991 Human Fertilisation & Embryology Act 1990: abortion and embryo research, the new law. Blackstone, London

■ Useful addresses

British Infertility Counselling Association
Eileen Brunton (Secretary)
Social Work Department
Simpson Maternity Pavilion
Lauriston Place
Edinburgh EH9 9YW

DI Network
PO Box 265
Sheffield S3 7YX

Human Fertilisation and Embryology Authority
Paxton House
30 Artillery Lane
London E1 7LS

ISSUE (The National Fertility Association)
509 Aldridge Road
Great Barr
Birmingham B44 8NA

Multiple Births Foundation
Queen Charlotte's & Chelsea Hospital
Goldhawk Road
London W6 0XG

NEEDS (National Egg and Embryo Donation Society)
The Regional IVF Unit
St Mary's Hospital
Manchester M3 0JH

TAMBA (Twins and Multiple Births Association)
PO Box 30
Little Sutton
South Wirral L66 1TH

Chapter 7

Women with learning disabilities: the midwife's role

Helen R. Minns

The Disabled Persons Act 1986, the Children Act 1989 and the National Health Service and Care in the Community Act 1990 place a responsibility on statutory providers to deliver services that reflect the rights, interests and needs of service users represented by themselves or by people advocating on their behalf (Gosling 1992).

These changes in legislation, together with a campaign to empower those with learning disabilities, are providing opportunities for couples to make choices about their lives, including their fertility.

There is a wealth of information on facilities and services for the physically disabled embarking upon parenthood, but little for those with learning disabilities. Most of the articles and research that make up the body of literature are written by health professionals in the field of learning disabilities or by sociologists and psychologists. There is a lack of literature by midwives on their role in supporting families in which one or both parents have a learning disability.

The reason for the lack of empirical research may be because people with learning disabilities differ so greatly in their abilities and needs that it may seem inappropriate to collect data. Sample sizes would inevitably be small at a local level, and a multicentre approach would be necessary. It is also likely that, until relatively recently, the needs of men and women with learning disabilities were ignored.

This chapter explores some of the issues surrounding parenthood for those with learning disabilities. The current literature is analysed and areas for further research identified in order to provide evidence to inform practice.

Booth and Booth (1993a) highlight some dangers of using the available research uncritically to inform policy and practice in this area. The parents who have been reported on have not been representative. They have been institutionalised, have had inadequate social support or have been selected from referrals to services, such as child protection agencies, as they have been experiencing serious difficulties. It would be a mistake to assume that research to date presents a true account of the limitations and potential of parents with learning disabilities. It should always be borne in mind that our understanding is confined to people who were born, brought up, have lived and had their children during a time of repressive treatment and widely pervasive discrimination.

■ **It is assumed that you are already aware of the following:**

● The principles of adult education;

● The organisation of local health services;

● The constituents and role of the primary health care team;

● The constituents and role of the community learning difficulty team;

● The 1959 Mental Health Act;

● The 1990 Community Care Act.

■ **Definitions**

There are considerable inconsistencies in the literature relating to the terms used to describe people with learning disabilities. 'Mental handicap', 'mental retardation', 'developmental disability' and 'learning disability' are all terms used by professionals. The term 'learning disability' will be used throughout this chapter; it will appear in italics where the original term used in the text under discussion has been replaced.

There is also some inconsistency in the way in which the degree of disability is described by some authors. Attard (1988) reminds us that the diagnosis of *learning disability* prior to the 1959 Mental Health Act does not necessarily equate with the present criteria.

People with a learning disability have, generally from birth, a difficulty of variable severity associated with a limitation of reasoning and comprehension skills to the extent that they are at a disadvantage in society. The more complex the demands made on an individual, the harder it will be for him or her to respond appropriately (Lindsey *et al* 1993).

Some authors define the degree of disability in terms of mild, moderate or severe, others in terms of intelligence quotient (IQ). *Learning disability* refers to IQ scores below 70 with concomitant poor social adaptation, both being evident before adulthood. Normal IQ scores range from 90 to 110. Although the accuracy of intelligence tests is often debated, a score of 70 is generally accepted to approximate to a cognitive mental age of about 9 years. This means that a person's level of knowledge and learning ability parallels those of a child of this age, not that he or she acts like a 9-year-old (Keltner & Tymchuk 1992).

People with a learning disability are in all other respects as different from each other as are the non-disabled population. Some, but not all, have other disabilities, such as cerebral palsy, visual and hearing problems, epilepsy and autism. Each of these associated conditions will affect the presentation and needs of the person, but the presence of a particular physical characteristic is of little help in determining the best approach to care (Lindsey *et al* 1993).

■ Incidence

The evidence shows that parenting by people with learning disabilities is not a new phenomenon and was probably more widespread in the past than has ever been officially recognised or acknowledged (Booth & Booth 1993).

Thornton (1994) writes that the absence of a national register means that demographic information is not easy to obtain. The 1989 Audit Commission Report, however, suggests that there are 124 000 adults in the UK who have a learning disability. These numbers indicate that 20 in every 1000 people are affected.

In the USA, it has been estimated that 3 per cent of the childbearing population have *learning disabilities*. This translates to approximately 120 000 babies born each year to US mothers with serious intellectual limitations (Keltner 1992).

■ Sex education

Craft and Craft (1978) highlighted the need for sex education for those who have *learning disabilities*. They experience many of the same feelings and drives as the rest of the population, but have commonly been left in ignorance on how to cope with them in a socially acceptable manner. Because a whole area of social education has been neglected, those with *learning disabilities* are all too likely to lack the skills that would give them some defence against exploitation and enable them to satisfy their social and sexual needs without bringing them into conflict with the law.

Kempton (1972) has noted some of the reasons why people with *learning disabilities* tend to have only partial and inaccurate knowledge about sexuality. They are often treated as perpetual children who have no interest in sexual matters; their peers (a source of information for normal youngsters) are likely to be equally ignorant, and they usually lack the degree of literacy necessary to find out for themselves from written sources.

Sex education has become a well-established part of the therapeutic and training regimes for people with learning disabilities. It is essential to give information about human sexuality and sexual behaviour.

Lindsay *et al* (1974) report on the evaluation of changes in client attitude towards relationships, following a 9-month sex education programme. The main purpose of such programmes is to increase sexual knowledge. An experimental group (46 adults: 26 men and 20 women) with a mild or moderate disability was compared with a control group (14 adults: 7 men and 7 women) in terms of acquisition of sexual knowledge. They were simply tested and retested 4 months later. Results showed that there was an increase in the number of correct responses given to questions about sexual knowledge by the group who received sex education but no increase in those of the control group who had received no sex education.

However, other aspects of sex education are equally important, and Lindsay *et al* (1994) analyse the changes in attitudes in clients following a sex education course. Personal confidence about one's own sexuality, self-image and attitudes towards sexuality are all likely to be discussed and reviewed during sessions. Changes in these aspects are harder to measure, especially as therapists and clients bring to the discussions their feelings, prejudices and values.

Lindsay *et al* (1994) used a sex education course based on material entitled 'Sexuality education for the lower functioning mentally handicapped' (Concord Films Council Ltd). The course includes basic information on parts of the male and female body, puberty, social interaction, sexuality and childbirth, birth control, sexually transmitted disease, parenting and marriage. This basic format is supplemented with sex education material from the Scottish Health Education Council.

Reviewing educational material and participating in some aspects of the sex education programme would be a first step towards midwives contributing to care for those with learning disabilities.

■ Integration of people with learning disabilities into the community

Normalisation is the process of making the lives of people with learning disabilities as close to those of mainstream society as possible (Wolfensberger 1972). There is a growing awareness of the needs of those with learning disabilities, particularly as they begin to become integrated into the community. Education of the general public, especially those living in the immediate neighbourhood, needs to continue, as prejudices still prevail.

Where couples are living in the community, it is essential that they have easy access to the health services, particularly to the members of the primary health care team. Parents, carers and practitioners in the community should have information about services available, including family planning, gynaecological and maternity services.

Rodgers (1994) explores the barriers to good primary health care for people with learning disabilities. She identifies a wide range of professionals who may be involved in their care. These include members of the primary health care team consisting of the GP, practice nurse, district nurse, midwife and health visitor.

The community learning difficulty team includes professionals with particular skills and experience in supporting people with learning disabilities. There is a core membership of a community mental handicap nurse and social worker, often supplemented by other specialist workers, such as speech therapists, occupational therapists, physiotherapists and psychologists.

Rodgers (1994) discusses interprofessional collaboration and its implications for good practice. She identifies the need for further work to improve the provision of care and assess users' experiences of the service. She also suggests that primary health care professionals may be unaware of the medical problems that are more common for people with learning disabilities.

Medical problems said to be more common in this group are hearing and visual disabilities, hypertension, chronic bronchitis, epilepsy, cerebral palsy, gross obesity, spinal deformities, skin disorders and mental health problems (Centre for Research and Information into Mental Disability 1990). There is also a need to be aware of the possibility of nutritional disorders, dental problems and 'polypharmacy', in which a range of medications is prescribed and not necessarily adequately monitored, as well as new health challenges, such as HIV and AIDS. People with Down's syndrome have unique health concerns, notably a higher incidence of thyroid disorders, atlanto-axial subluxation and Alzheimer's disease (Rubin 1987).

The primary health care team has an important role in health promotion for all those registered with the health centre. Helping couples with learning disabilities to become more conscious of their health needs requires sensitivity and an understanding of their particular circumstances. A key worker may be identified to ensure that a woman has appropriate advice on such matters as sexual health, including cervical cytology, the prevention of sexually transmitted diseases and contraception.

■ Preconception care and advice

'Learning disability' is a term used to encompass a wide variation of ability. Couples either thinking of or actually embarking on a pregnancy should have the best possible advice and support from health professionals in relation to their individual circumstances and needs.

The rights of people with learning disabilities has been a contentious issue since the early 1900s, particularly in relation to their fertility and its control. Greer (1984) describes the history of eugenics and the formation of the Eugenics Society, which explored ways in which the physical and mental quality of a people could be controlled and improved by selective breeding.

Nowadays, more people with learning disabilities have the opportunity to make choices about their lives in general, particularly about their fertility. Choices of contraception should be based upon the couple's requirements and ability to use the method, rather than on other people's opinions of their needs (Lister 1994).

Chaplin (1992) writes about the 'circles of support' concept, which was first developed by Judith Snow and Marsha Forest in Toronto, Canada, in 1980 but is not widely known in the UK. Essentially, a circle of support is a group of people coming together to help the person with the disability accomplish certain personal visions or goals that he or she would be unable to accomplish alone. Circle members are usually friends, family members, co-workers, neighbours, church members and sometimes service providers. The majority are unpaid; they are there because they care about the focus person and make a commitment to work on his or her behalf. This support when a couple are contemplating parenthood would be invaluable.

Where there is the opportunity to explore the options relating to the possible outcomes of pregnancy, it would be preferable to do this during the preconception period. Unfortunately, the reality is that many pregnancies occur before such planning can take place.

In order to make an informed choice, the couple contemplating pregnancy will want to know the likely incidence of handicap in the offspring. In a literature review on risk of handicap in offspring, Attard (1988) reported on the results of a study by Reed and Reed (1965). At the Institute of Human Genetics, they looked at the records of 7728 children. In 89 cases where both parents had an IQ under 70, 40 per cent of the children were classified as educationally retarded (IQ at 74). When only one parent had an IQ below 70, 15 per cent of children were educationally retarded, with 54 per cent of the children having an IQ above 90. Of 7035 children with neither parent retarded, 1 per cent had an IQ less than 70. They calculated that for a mentally handicapped person with an IQ under 70, the expectation for one of their children also to score an IQ under 70 was 17.1 per cent (Attard 1988).

Curtis (Chapter 2 in this volume) and Spedding *et al* (1995) discuss the importance of health prior to and around the time of conception. Those with learning disabilities are no different from any couple planning a pregnancy. When planning a pregnancy, it is recommended that the woman changes from oral contraception or the intrauterine device, to barrier or natural methods of contraception. This may not be practical as both methods require motivation and planning, which may present difficulties where one or both partners have a learning disability.

■ Antenatal care

As soon as the pregnancy has been diagnosed, referral to the maternity services should be made, usually by the GP to the midwife. Women with learning disabilities, in the absence of medical conditions, are at no greater risk of complications of pregnancy than is any other woman. Antenatal care should be carried out by the midwife. Referral can be made to the consultant obstetric department if complications arise.

An initial visit to the woman's own home, where the woman is most likely to feel confident, is beneficial to establish the relationship. In any family, it is not only the mother and father who are involved in parenting: grandparents, aunts and other members of the family, or friends, are important and should be involved in the health education so that the mother is not confused by conflicting advice. It is also a chance to meet those who provide support on a daily basis and involve them in the care planning. The importance of written communications between professionals and family to co-ordinate care is discussed by Rose (1994).

Woman-centred care is one of the fundamental principles of good practice (DoH 1993). It will be vital for the woman with learning disabilities to maintain a feeling of being in control. Continuity of care and carer throughout the antenatal, intrapartum and postpartum periods is preferable, and every effort should be made to minimise the number of midwives involved.

Most maternity services now encourage women to carry their own case notes. Notes should be personalised, and woman-centred care can only be achieved if the notes are written from the mother's point of view (Magill-Cuerden 1992). This is particularly important for women with learning disabilities. In some circumstances, where the mother is unable to read, the use of pictorial illustrations will be an appropriate addition to the more formal records of examinations and discussions.

Even people with a milder disability may find it difficult to understand long words, abstract ideas, comparisons and other complexities of language. A normal tone of voice and simple language should be used. It is wise to avoid comparisons between the human body and plumbing, or explanations based on a knowledge of human biology. Euphemisms should also be avoided, and it is better to use words such as 'hurt' or 'sore' rather than 'tender' and 'discomfort'. Medical jargon and abbreviations should be avoided. The names of parts of the body may not be known, and pictures might be used to check that the meaning is clear. It is important to be aware that those with *learning disabilities* may have a short attention span and need information to be repeated several times (Lindsey *et al* 1993).

Because of lack of access to prenatal care in the past, women with *learning disabilities* have had increased problems with pregnancy complications, such as elevated blood pressure, proteinuria, anaemia, poor weight gain, preterm labour and infections (Carty *et al* 1993). It would be interesting to collect the data on complications of pregnancy as access to care improves.

Carty *et al* (1993) suggest that adults with *learning disabilities* are often unaware of signs and symptoms of illness, so do not know when to seek health care. Listing signs and symptoms of common problems, such as infection and preterm labour, on an index card taped to the refrigerator may help the woman with *learning disabilities* to remember to call the midwife. Adding numbers for the ambulance, hospital, fire and police services to this card would also be helpful (Carty *et al* 1993). However, it is possible that this approach may create more anxiety than is necessary. Knowing how to contact carers, who will ask appropriate questions, may be more effective and supportive.

Turk and Brown (1993) report on a survey on the incidence of sexual abuse in adults with learning disabilities. Physical abuse is known to cause learning disabilities in some circumstances, and Groce (1988) estimates that as many as 1 in 10 children with learning disabilities may have acquired their disability as a direct result of physical assault or neglect. Similarly, learning disability as a consequence of an incestuous union has been well documented (Jancar & Johnston 1990).

The pregnancy may, therefore, have occurred as a result of rape or sexual abuse, and this needs to be handled in a sensitive way by practitioners experienced in this area. Courtois and Courtois Riley (1992) describe the need for extra sensitivity and awareness on the part of midwives when a woman recalls her abuse or when pregnancy or labour stimulates memories. Most important, caregivers must not dismiss reports of abuse and/or downplay its past or current significance for the woman. Ignorance, denial and even hostility toward reports of abuse by caregivers have all been reported by survivors. Such responses can result in a second psychological injury because they are given by an authority figure in a helping profession that is expected to understand or, at the very least, respond with sensitivity. It is particularly important for midwives to be sensitive when caring for a woman with learning disabilities.

■ Preparation for parenthood – antenatal education

Although antenatal education on a one-to-one basis may be necessary, it is also important for the couple to meet with others who are pregnant. There is a danger of social isolation, and group support is one of the benefits of antenatal classes.

Classes with an informal approach to antenatal education may be the most appropriate. Women with learning disabilities share many of the problems experienced by young, single mothers. Poverty, unemployment, housing difficulties, victimisation and inadequate skills in forming and maintaining relationships are all commonly experienced by both these groups (Minns 1989).

Preparation for the birth will need to be carried out at a level appropriate to the woman's needs. A variety of teaching methods should be used. If the delivery is to take place in hospital, a visit to a ward and a delivery room on several occasions will help the couple to become familiar with the surroundings. Demonstrations of baby bathing, nappy changing and learning to hold a newborn baby will all help in the learning process.

There are few leaflets written for the woman with learning difficulties; *Pregnancy and the disabled woman* is one leaflet written by a midwife (Rotheram 1989). Although written for the physically disabled, there is a useful checklist on getting pregnant, care during pregnancy, during and after delivery, with advice, help and information. The leaflet has been written as a result of a research study individually interviewing eight women with restricted mobility. The study was undertaken to identify the family health care and childbirth services that are available to women with physical disabilities. It also identifies deficiencies in the service and makes recommendations for improvements.

Although this is a study involving physically disabled women, it highlighted the need for health care professionals to change their attitudes in order to bring the subject of pregnancy and the disabled into the open. A similar study would be useful for planning a strategy for the provision of maternity care for those with learning disabilities.

Cross (1994) writes about the care of Ms White, a 32-year-old woman with a mild learning disability. Cross describes her role as community nurse of the learning disability team in supporting a couple throughout the pregnancy and enabling them to gain in confidence and ability. She describes the limited choice of teaching resources for use with couples with a learning disability. Cross (1994) used the Two-Can Resource Unit series designed for people with hearing loss. This comprises simple short word captions and pictures describing the procedures at the antenatal clinic, in relaxation classes and during labour, and a section was discussed at each session.

☐ **Intrapartum care**

Labour is an anxious time for most couples, and for a woman who may have limited understanding of the birth processes, it can be particularly stressful.

Familiarity with the place of birth and the midwife who will care for the couple can do much to allay the couple's fears. In some situations, a home birth may be most appropriate, particularly if there is good family support. Early discharge after delivery in hospital might be another alternative.

Simple explanations as labour progresses are important. A familiar voice using the same words as were used to describe labour during antenatal sessions also helps to reassure the couple.

Examinations, such as vaginal examinations, should be kept to a minimum and conducted with special care. Full explanations of procedures should be given beforehand.

It is especially important where labour does not progress normally that the obsteric team works together to ensure that the woman feels safe. This situation highlights the benefits of having the same midwife, already known to the couple, continuing to provide care throughout labour.

Abuse survivors might use familiar defences such as dissociation ('going away') to cope with physical and psychological pain. Flashbacks to abuse brought on by labour and birth may inadvertently expose the woman to memories of events related to the original trauma. Midwives can expect such reactions and be prepared to give verbal encouragement to the woman to stay in the present, to assure her of safety and to distinguish past from present (Courtois & Courtois Riley 1992).

Enabling the couple to debrief after the birth is an important part of the psychological care and may take many months. It will be an important role for the midwife in the postnatal period and should be continued by the health visitor.

There is little written about intrapartum care for couples with learning disabilities. It is an area that requires further investigation to produce guidelines for good practice.

■ **Postnatal support**

Continuity of care and carer is as important in the postnatal period as it is in pregnancy or labour. Midwives, carers and relatives need to work together to enable the woman to recover from the birth both physically and emotionally. Teaching the range of skills needed to care for the baby will require time and patience.

Rose (1994) describes the care of a woman who had *learning disabilities* and suffered from familial microcephaly. As their health visitor, Rose was able to work with the couple using a problem solving approach to overcome the difficulties of feeding a preterm baby. The baby had been delivered by caesarean section at 37 weeks gestation, weighing just over 4 lb, and there was some concern over the baby's failure to gain weight. There appeared to be a discrepancy between the recorded amount of milk taken and the baby's weight gain. The mother was unable to calculate the difference between the amount of milk offered and the amount taken. A cardboard calculator was devised, which the mother could stand next to the feeding bottle and use to read off the amount of milk left.

It would seem that, if it were possible, encouraging the woman to breastfeed would be more effective in reducing the complications of preparation and measurements involved in artificial feeding. Carty *et al* (1993) identify the infants of mothers with *learning disabilities* to be at risk of dehydration, gastroenteritis and/or failure to thrive. Equally important in promoting breastfeeding would be the satisfaction experienced by the mother and the increase in her own self-esteem as a result of successfully feeding her baby.

Keltner (1992) conducted a study aimed to determine the caregiving deficits of mothers who have *learning disabilities*, to measure how the variance of the mother's intellectual abilities contributes to caregiving outcomes (child health and development) and to explore what naturally occurring caregiving supports or substitutes contribute to the health of infants of mothers with intellectual limitations. A prospective non-experimental study design was employed using two groups of mothers with different intellectual abilities. Group A consisted of 34 women with IQs below 75. Group B comprised 18 women with IQs above 85. It was conducted in the southern USA, an area where poverty is particularly marked. Efforts were made to match the groups for age, race and parity, and all were of low income. The mothers were recruited from prenatal clinics, school pregnancy programmes and hospitals. All had monthly home visits. There were some difficulties due to the small sample size.

Keltner's study identified the need for mothers with *learning disabilities* to have professional caring to support their role. The deficits identified were lack of functional skills such as infant feeding. Although no statistically significant differences were found between the health of the children in either group, three of the children of mothers with IQs below 75 experienced growth and developmental deficits. It is possible that significant differences may have been found with a larger sample. Mothers with IQs below 75 generally perceived themselves as being less competent than did those with IQs over 85, although one mother with a learning disability assigned herself the highest value for perceived competence. This highlights the need for assessing perceptions of caregiving competence in order to communicate more clearly with mothers with learning disabilities.

Inadequate maternal–child interaction was also identified and indicates a serious caregiving need for mothers with learning disabilities. Maternal–child interaction is fundamental to many important outcomes of care, including the cognitive development of children. This is the probable mechanism through which *learning disabilities* are passed from generation to generation. Keltner (1992) identified maternal–child interaction as an area in which further studies are necessary.

Niven (1992) discusses families in which there are actual or potential difficulties in parent–infant interaction; these could also be applied to some parents with learning disabilities. Niven (1992) describes interventions based on the Brazelton Neonatal Behavioural Assessment Scheme (BNBAS) that have been used to enhance the parents' perception of the newborn as an interesting social being. The BNBAS is an interactive assessment that reveals the complexities and competences of the newborn (Woroby 1985).

By demonstrating that the baby has some impressive abilities and that he or she can interact with adults, this assessment makes it obvious to the parents that they have a baby who is an individual human being capable of responding to their overtures, rather than a passive, helpless, boring creature who just needs to be fed and changed and does nothing but sleep and cry. Although administering the BNBAS requires specialist training, the principles of its use can be used as an aid to improving parents' appreciation of the capabilities of their child. Midwives might find it a useful approach in the postnatal period.

Social support appears to be fundamental to the ability of those with learning disabilities to cope with parenting skills (personal observation). Friends and family may fulfil this role, or alternatives may have to be found. Childminders are an underused resource that can help to keep families together (Randall 1995).

An initiative has been set up by the National Childminding Association and funded by Children in Need to create a community childminding scheme. The childminders could be used where parents have special needs, including *learning disabilities*. The ultimate purpose is to keep children out of care, to help families overcome or cope with whatever barriers there are to caring for their children and to keep them together. In many cases, the scheme will provide a few hours respite care each day or week (Carrington 1995).

George (1994) describes a programme for parents with learning disabilities, called the Special Parenting Service, run by the Cornwall and Isles of Scilly Learning Disabilities NHS Trust. The Trust now organises and runs specialist assessments for social services departments, the courts and others; this also involves specialist teaching of parents and weekly parents' group meetings. The Service trains staff and takes a central role in multiagency co-ordination and programme planning. Booklets, audio-tapes and a videotape have been produced. The service's preventive work is not just in teaching specific skills but is also designed to be empowering for the individual and family. It uses co-operative rather than coercive teaching methods. Great emphasis is placed on the continuity of staff–parent relationships.

Booth and Booth (1993b) identify general lessons for practitioners: when working with parents, look for strengths and positive qualities of families (and how they can be reinforced), rather than just for their weaknesses: explore practical ways of reducing the pressures on the family from environmental threats, thus lightening the parenting load; be ready to respond to the early signs of stress instead of waiting for the crisis to occur; and ensure that the parents have access to independent, informed and sympathetic advice whenever issues relating to parental responsibilities and the care of children arise.

Andron and Tymchuk (1987) predict that we may have to wait until a whole generation of people has lived in the community before we can begin fully to appreciate their qualities as parents.

■ Recommendations for clinical practice in the light of currently available evidence

1. There is a need for research to establish the numbers of babies born to mothers with learning difficulties.

2. There is a need for the continuing collection of data nationally to evaluate service provision for those parents with learning difficulties.

3. An evaluation of the parents' experiences of the maternity services should be undertaken, with recommendations for improvements.

4. An evaluation of the cost implications of supporting parents with learning disabilities in the community should be carried out.

■ Practice check

- Have you had study sessions on the special needs of mothers with learning disabilities? The community learning disability team would be a useful resource to facilitate this.

- Do you know how many couples with learning disabilities are being supported in the community in which you work?

- Evaluate the experience of families in which one or both parents have a learning disability. Set standards in relation to maternity care for mothers with learning disabilities and regularly reassess the quality of care.

- Examine your feelings and attitudes towards couples with learning disabilities becoming parents and your role in supporting them.

- Does your local maternity or health education unit have a range of audiovisual aids available for educating couples with special learning needs about pregnancy, childbirth and parenting skills?

- Consider the issue of consent to treatment for adults in relation to those with learning disabilities and your responsibilities where there are significant ethical or moral concerns.

☐ Acknowledgements

I would like to thank Janet McCray, Principal Lecturer, University of Portsmouth, for her help in the preparation of this chapter.

■ References

Andron L, Tymchuk A 1987 Parents who are mentally retarded. In Craft A (ed.) Mental handicap and sexuality: issues and perspectives. DJ Costello, Tunbridge Wells, Ch 11, p238–58

Attard M 1988 Mentally handicapped parents – some issues to consider in relation to pregnancy. British Journal of Mental Subnormality 34(66): 3–9

Audit Commission 1989 Developing community care for adults with a mental handicap. Occasional Paper No 9. HMSO, London

Booth T, Booth W 1993a Parenting with learning difficulties: lessons for practitioners. British Journal of Social Work 23: 459–80

Booth T, Booth W 1993b Power to parents. Nursing Times 89(35): 61–3

Carrington L (1995) The minders. Community Care 1061: 25

Carty E, Conine T, Holbrook A, Riddell L 1993 Childbearing and parenting with a disability or chronic illness. Midwifery Today 28: 17–19, 40–2

Centre for Research and Information into Mental Disability (CRIMD) 1990 Primary Health Care for People with Learning Disability. Policy Paper No 1. CRIMD, University of Birmingham

Chaplin J 1992 Making ties and connections: integrating people with disabilities and learning difficulties into the community. Community Health Action 24: 7–8

Children Act 1989 HMSO, London

Courtois C, Courtois Riley C (1992) Pregnancy and childbirth as triggers for abuse memories: implications for care. Birth 19: 222–3

Craft M, Craft A 1978 Sex and the mentally handicapped. Routledge & Kegan Paul, London

Cross G 1994 The right to choose. Nursing Times 90(39): 60–2

Department of Health 1993 Changing childbirth. Report of the Expert Maternity Group HMSO, London

Disabled Persons Act 1986 HMSO, London

George M 1994 Whose difficulty is it anyway? Community Care 1026: 26–7

Gosling J 1992 Involving people with disabilities in planning services. Journal of the National Community Health Resource Community Health Action 24: 5–6

Greer G 1984 Eugenics. Sex and destiny, the politics of human fertility. Secker & Warburg, London, Ch 10, p255–94

Groce N E 1988 Special groups at risk of abuse: the disabled. In Straus MB (ed.) Abuse and victimisation across the lifespan. Johns Hopkins University Press, New York, Ch 12, p223–9

Jancar J, Johnston SJ 1990 Incest and mental handicap. Journal of Mental Deficiency Research 34: 483–90

Keltner B 1992 Caregiving by mothers with mental retardation. Family and Community Health 15(2): 10–18

Keltner B, Tymchuk A 1992 Reaching out to mothers with mental retardation. MCN The American Journal of Maternal/Child Nursing 17(3): 136–40

Kempton W 1972 Guidelines for planning a training course on human sexuality and the retarded. Philadelphia: Planned Parenthood Association of SE Pennsylvania. Cited in Craft A, Craft M 1983 Sex education and counselling for mentally handicapped people. Costello, Tunbridge Wells, p13

Lindsay WR, Michie AM, Staines C, Bellshaw E, Culross G 1994 Client attitudes towards relationships: changes following a sex education programme. British Journal of Learning Disabilities 22: 70–3

Lindsey M, Singh K, Perrett A 1993 Management of learning disability in the general hospital. British Journal of Hospital Medicine 50(4): 182–6

Lister KD 1994 National Association of Family Planning Nurses Journal 26: 86–94

Magill-Cuerden J 1992 A question of communication. Modern Midwife 2(6): 4–5

Mental Health Act 1959 HMSO, London

Minns HR 1989 Young mum's club. Nursing Times 85(28): 68–9

National Health Service and Community Care Act 1990 HMSO, London, Ch 19

Niven CA 1992 Psychological care for families before, during and after birth. Butterworth–Heinemann, Oxford

Randall L 1995 Cited in Carrington L, The minders. Community Care 1061: 5

Reed EW, Reed SC 1965 Mental retardation: a family study. WB Saunders, Philadelphia

Rodgers J 1994 Primary health care provision for people with learning disabilities. Health and Social Care in the Community 2(1): 11–17

Rose V 1994 Health education for parents with special needs. Health Visitor 67(3): 95–6

Rotheram J 1989 Care of the disabled woman during pregnancy. Nursing Standard 4(10): 36–9

Rubin L 1987 Health care needs of adults with mental retardation. Mental Retardation 25(4): 201–6

Spedding S, Wilson J, Wright S, Jackson A 1995 Nutrition for pregnancy and lactation In Alexander J, Levy V, Roch S (eds) Aspects of midwifery practice: a research-based approach. Macmillan, Basingstoke, Ch 1, p1–23

Thornton C 1994 Primary planning. Nursing Times   90(12): 65–6

Turk V, Brown H 1993 The sexual abuse of adults with learning disabilities: results of a two year incidence survey. Mental Handicap Research   6(3): 193–216

Wolfensberger W 1972 The principle of normalisation in human services. National Institute on Mental Retardation, Toronto

Woroby J 1985 A review of Brazelton based interventions to enhance parent–infant interaction. Journal of Reproductive Infant Psychology   3: 64–74. Cited in Niven CA 1992 Psychological care for families before, during and after birth. Butterworth–Heinemann, Oxford, p64–74

■ Suggested further reading

Journal of Disability, Pregnancy and Parenthood International, Arrowhead Publications, 51 Thames Village, London W4 3UF

McGaw S 1995 What's it like to be a parent? Book One in the Parenting Series. Available from the British Institute of Learning Disabilities, Wolverhampton Road, Kidderminster, Worcs DY10 3PP

■ Useful addresses

BILD Current Awareness Service
British Institute of Learning Disabilities
Wolverhampton Road
Kidderminster
Worcs DY10 3PP

Disability Group
Maternity Alliance
15 Britannia Street
London WC1X 9JP

Disability Alliance
88–94 Universal House
Wentworth Street
London E1 7SA

Two-Can Resource Unit
Teaching Material Nos 14 (Antenatal Clinics), 19 (Relaxation) and 20 (Labour). Available from Rycote Centre for the Deaf, Derby DE1 3HF

Chapter 8

Pre-eclampsia

Tansy M. Cheston

Pre-eclampsia has been known by various names in the past, some of them still in use. The Victorians knew it as 'toxaemia of pregnancy' because they thought it was caused by one or more poisons circulating in the mother's bloodstream. This term is now obsolete, although a later description – 'pre-eclamptic toxaemia' – persists, mostly because it can be conveniently abbreviated to PET.

Pre-eclampsia is recognised as a syndrome, that is, a cluster of typical features that have to occur together before the diagnosis can be made. Unfortunately, there is no specific diagnostic test, which would be a more accurate way of making the diagnosis. The cluster usually comprises new hypertension (that is, the diastolic pressure reaching or exceeding 90 mmHg after previously lower readings) and new proteinuria (at least one plus on dipstick testing, consistently present in every sample tested in the absence of a urinary tract infection), with or without oedema. 'Pregnancy-induced hypertension' (PIH) and 'hypertensive disease of pregnancy' are names given to the sign of raised blood pressure alone. Both terms are often, but incorrectly, used as alternative names for pre-eclampsia, although they refer merely to transient hypertension without proteinuria appearing at the end of pregnancy. Such isolated hypertension may just as easily reflect chronic hypertension revealed for the first time in pregnancy as the more threatening pre-eclampsia, in which the hypertension is associated with persistent proteinuria.

This chapter will discuss the risks for the mother and fetus, the aetiology and incidence of pre-eclampsia and eclampsia, signs, symptoms, diagnosis, complications and suggested recommendations for clinical practice in the light of currently available evidence.

■ **It is assumed that you are already aware of the following:**

- The basic anatomy and physiology of the pregnant woman;

- Fetoplacental physiology;
- Routine antenatal care.

■ Risks to mother and fetus

Pre-eclampsia is a serious hazard for both mother and fetus. The risks to the mother include cerebral haemorrhage, eclamptic convulsions, pulmonary oedema, hepatic and renal impairment, disseminated intravascular coagulation and death. Hypertensive disease of pregnancy, which includes pre-eclampsia, is still the major cause of maternal mortality in England and Wales (DoH 1994).

The risks to the fetus are those of placental insufficiency – intrauterine growth retardation, asphyxia, abruptio placentae and intrauterine death. The neonate suffers particularly from the consequences of preterm delivery, particularly with respiratory distress syndrome, and also from polycythaemia and hypoglycaemia.

■ Detection by screening

Pre-eclampsia has two key characteristics that make it very difficult to detect and manage. First, it is largely a 'silent' disease, which in most cases causes no symptoms of illness at all until the later stages. Thus it can only be reliably detected by screening checks – regular repetitive searches for tell-tale signs during pregnancy. Second, pre-eclampsia always gets progressively worse as the pregnancy continues, although at different rates in different women. Nothing as yet can be done to halt and reverse this relentless progress; ultimately, the only treatment is to deliver the baby, which guarantees complete recovery of the mother in the vast majority of cases, although pregnancy can sometimes be prolonged for a short while, with close monitoring, to gain fetal maturity.

■ Eclampsia

Eclampsia is the occurrence of convulsions in association with signs of pre-eclampsia. In 1992, the British Eclampsia Survey Team (BEST; Douglas & Redman 1994) measured the incidence of eclampsia and its maternal and perinatal mortality. They found that eclampsia complicates nearly 1 in 2000 pregnancies in the UK; nearly 1 in 50 affected women dies, as does 1 in 14 of their offspring. It may present unheralded by warning signs.

Although most cases occur during or after delivery at term, those that develop preterm (less than 37 weeks gestation) and before delivery seemed to be particularly severe (Douglas & Redman 1994). Eclampsia is just one of a number of endstage crises that can strike the pre-eclamptic woman or her unborn baby. The HELLP syndrome (see below) is another, one just as dangerous and probably more common.

■ Incidence of pre-eclampsia

The incidence is:

- 1 in 10 in primigravidae;
- 1 in 20 in multigravidae.

■ Aetiology of pre-eclampsia

The pathogenesis of pre-eclampsia is complex and still incompletely understood. We know that the primary pathology is localised within the gravid uterus, as the condition resolves after delivery. The cause must lie in the placenta as the disorder is specific to pregnancy, but it can occur in the absence of a fetus, as with hydatidiform mole, when the uterus contains only disordered placental tissue (Page 1938; Scott 1958).

The disease is associated with inadequate adaptation of the maternal circulation to the placenta. In normal pregnancy, the endarteries that deliver maternal blood into the intervillous space – the spiral arteries – are remodelled (and enlarged) in two stages to permit the vastly expanded blood flow that the placenta needs (DeWolf *et al* 1980). The first stage of remodelling, involving the decidual segments of the spiral arteries, is normally complete by the end of the first trimester; the second, involving myometrial segments, is fully developed just before mid-term (Robertson *et al* 1975; Pijenborg *et al* 1981).

The remodelling is carried out by cells of the placenta itself – cytotrophoblast cells – which detach themselves from the main body of the placenta and invade the underlying maternal tissues of the placental bed, including the spiral arteries. In pre-eclampsia, it has been demonstrated that the second wave of cytotrophoblastic invasion (that occurring early in the second trimester) is inhibited, so that the myometrial segments of the spiral arteries fail to dilate (Fig. 8.1). They retain their musculoelastic structure and smaller calibre, and when examined at

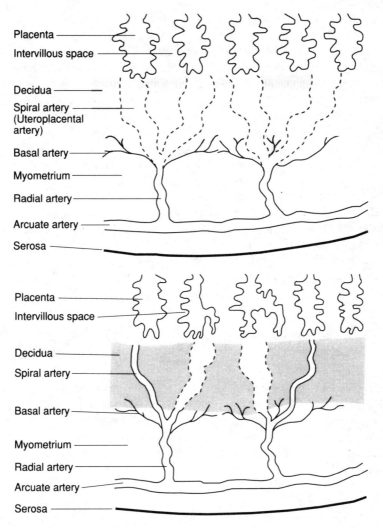

Figure 8.1 (a) Diagram of normal blood supply to the placenta. Note the termination of the radial arteries each into two spiral arteries which have been physiologically converted (dashed). For clarity, the marked coiling and distension have not been drawn. (b) Diagram of abnormal blood supply to the placenta. Note physiological changes (dashed) in some decidual segments of spiral arteries but absent in others. Myometrial segments are drawn without physiological changes, as in pre-eclampsia, but these segments may show physiological changes in some cases with small-for-gestational-age infants. (Reproduced from Khong *et al* 1986, with permission from the authors, The British Journal of Obstetrics and Gynaecology and Blackwell Science Publishers.)

delivery lack the usual remnants of infiltrating cytotrophoblast (Brosens *et al* 1972; Robertson *et al* 1975; Gerretsen *et al* 1981). They are thus too small to deliver the bloodflow needed by the third trimester placenta.

There is thus inadequate uteroplacental blood flow and placental hypoxia, and it is thought that this is the underlying problem in pre-eclampsia. The poor placental blood supply and flow of nutrients and oxygen explain the fetal growth retardation. However, the diverse features of the maternal syndrome (hypertension, proteinuria, disseminated intra-vascular coagulation, hepatic dysfunction and convulsions) require a different explanation.

Until recently, it was difficult to formulate a unifying hypothesis for the role of the placenta in pre-eclampsia. A possible answer is that the maternal syndrome is the end result of diffuse maternal endothelial dysfunction caused directly or indirectly by a circulating factor originating from the ischaemic placenta (Roberts *et al* 1989; Roberts & Redman 1993). The endothelium controls arterial tone, so that the hypertension of pre-eclampsia, thought to be due to increased peripheral resistance (Groenedijik *et al* 1984), can be explained by spasm resulting from an imbalance of the endothelial controlling mechanisms. Intense localised vasoconstrictions, resulting in ischaemia, which is thought to be the primary cause of convulsions (eclampsia) and liver damage (Sheehan *et al* 1973), probably share the same origins, that is, endothelial cell damage. The latter can also cause increased vascular permeability, with leakage of protein into the urine, loss of fluid from the vascular compartment into the surrounding tissues (oedema) and an associated fall in plasma volume (Gallery *et al* 1979, 1981).

These ideas concerning the origins of pre-eclampsia lead to a two-stage model of the disease: stage 1 (inadequate remodelling of the spiral arteries) is preclinical and without symptoms, whereas stage 2 (diffuse maternal endothelial cell damage) manifests itself as the maternal and fetal syndromes (Redman 1993).

■ Risk factors

First-time mothers are several times more prone to pre-eclampsia than are those in second or subsequent pregnancies. There is some evidence that it is pregnancy by the present partner (primipaternity) rather than first pregnancy itself (primiparity) that is important (Robillard *et al* 1994). Unfortunately, however, it is not true that after suffering pre-eclampsia in a first pregnancy, a woman will not get it again (Campbell & MacGillivray 1985). The predisposition to pre-eclampsia may be inherited (Cooper & Liston 1979), so that a positive maternal family history is a risk factor: the daughters of eclamptic women are eight times more likely to have pre-eclampsia than would be expected for the general population (Chesley *et al* 1968). Pre-eclamptic women also tend to be shorter than average (Baird 1977). Predisposing fetal factors include multiple pregnancy (MacGillivray 1959), hydatidiform mole (Chun *et al*

1964), hydrops fetalis with or without rhesus isoimmunisation (Jeffcoate & Scott 1959), fetal triploidy and fetal trisomy 13 (Boyd *et al* 1987).

Maternal medical conditions, such as renal disease, diabetes, chronic hypertension, migraine and autoimmune disease, all predispose to pre-eclampsia. Other factors include increasing maternal age, especially over the age of 35 years, and teenage pregnancies (Redman 1995).

■ How to detect pre-eclampsia

Pre-eclampsia can occur at any time in the second half of pregnancy and must be detected in the symptomless woman by screening for its signs. One of the most critical aspects of screening for pre-eclampsia is the interval between antenatal checks. This is difficult to standardise because the disease has an extremely variable speed of progression, some cases developing over months and others reaching danger levels with unnerving speed. In cases of so-called fulminating pre-eclampsia, the mother and her doctors are confronted with a raging crisis, which has evolved from nothing in the space of a week or two, sometimes even less. An interval of more than 2 weeks, or even more than 1 week between checks, can allow such crises to develop undetected.

In the UK there is no standard practice, but a typical programme for pregnant women is antenatal checks at 20, 24 and 28 weeks, then every 2 weeks until 36 weeks, and then weekly to full term. However, this leaves two potentially dangerous month-long gaps between 20 and 28 weeks in which early onset pre-eclampsia can escape detection; this is why disasters including maternal deaths occur more often during this critical period (DoH 1994). Towards term, with the increased frequency of visits, there is reason to believe that the current system of care works well, and most crises are thereby prevented. Those which occur are the ones with atypically fast presentations.

In 1992, BEST (Douglas & Redman 1994) measured the incidence of eclampsia, established how often it is preceded by signs of pre-eclampsia, documented the morbidity associated with eclampsia and determined the maternal case fatality rates. A prospective, descriptive study of every case of eclampsia in the UK in 1992 was collated from reviews of hospital case notes and questionnaires to general practitioners. All 279 hospitals in the UK with consultant obstetric units were included. Obstetricians and midwives notified 582 possible cases, of which 383 were confirmed as eclampsia. The national incidence of eclampsia was 4.9 per 10 000 maternities (Douglas & Redman 1994).

It was noted that of the 383 women, 325 (85 per cent) had been seen by a doctor or midwife in the week before their first convulsion. Eleven per cent had no recorded hypertension or proteinuria, 10 per cent had proteinuria but no hypertension, 22 per cent had hypertension alone, and 57 per cent of women had both proteinuria and hypertension at the final antenatal visit.

☐ **Antenatal tests**

Until such time as pre-eclampsia is more fully understood, it must, as has already been mentioned, remain a 'syndrome' recognised not by a unique causal agent but by a collection of characteristics and symptoms, which can each have other causes when considered individually but usually indicate pre-eclampsia when they occur together.

Once the pattern of antenatal care has been determined, four basic tests need to be repeated at each visit to detect warning signs of pre-eclampsia:

1. Blood pressure measurement;

2. Weight check;

3. Urine testing for protein;

4. Assessment of the baby's growth.

At least two signs must be present before the diagnosis can be made. Symptoms may also occur and should be checked for.

☐ **Blood pressure measurement**

Blood pressure levels are influenced by age, sex, race, body build and many other factors, particularly the circumstances in which the measurement is taken. Pregnant women are relatively young and usually fit. The range of blood pressures will therefore tend to be narrower than in the general population and distributed around mean levels that change at different stages of gestation but which in mid-pregnancy are lower than for a comparable non-pregnant population.

Blood pressure measurements should be made with the cuff at the level of the heart. If it is above or below this position, the pressure in the brachial artery will fall or rise because of hydrostatic forces. Posture should always be standardised, for example to the sitting position. Phase I of the Korotkoff sounds (clear tapping sounds) defines the systolic pressure and phase V (extinction of the Korotkoff sounds) is the diastolic endpoint (Shennan *et al* 1995); these two points should be used when recording measurements.

It is generally agreed that hypertension in obese individuals is over-diagnosed if a cuff is used which is too small in relation to the patient's arm circumference. If the arm circumference is over 35 cm, a cuff larger than the regular size should be used.

Although a rise in blood pressure is usually the first sign of pre-eclampsia, it is an unreliable one, partly because blood pressure is naturally variable with alternating 'highs' and 'lows', and partly because the measurement technique itself is rather crude and inaccurate. One high reading alone is not necessarily significant: the readings must be consistently raised. The actual level of blood pressure is probably less important than the amount by which it has risen above a 'baseline measurement' taken in early pregnancy. Any reading 25–30 mmHg higher than the baseline measurement should be taken seriously – the systolic figure is as important in this respect as the diastolic figure (Redman 1989).

□ **Weight check**

Oedema is probably the most confusing of all possible signs for pre-eclampsia because it is a common physiological feature of pregnancy. However, swelling is suspicious if it is associated with weight gain of more than 1 kg (2.2 lb) per week, with oedema of the face and hands, particularly if the blood pressure is raised. Excessive weight gain can be the first noticeable symptom of pre-eclampsia, but this can only be detected if regular weight checks are made at the antenatal visit, so that an emerging trend can be seen. Excessive weight gain may reflect 'hidden' fluid retention, such as early ascites (Abitbol 1969). Continuity in the weighing scales used is preferable.

□ **Proteinuria**

Proteinuria is the conventionally recognised but late sign of renal involvement in pre-eclampsia. Once present, it indicates a poorer prognosis for both mother and fetus than when it is absent (Butler & Bonham 1963; Naeye and Friedman 1979; Taylor *et al* 1954). On average, it appears about 3 weeks before intrauterine death or mandatory delivery (Redman *et al* 1976). A common error is to underestimate the importance of testing for proteinuria. This is an unacceptable omission because proteinuria can accompany only a slightly raised blood pressure or even predate a rise in the blood pressure (Douglas & Redman 1994). A reading of one plus protein on two or more occasions is a reason for admission to hospital, particularly if it is associated with any other signs of pre-eclampsia (Highby *et al* 1994).

☐ Intrauterine growth retardation

Poor fetal growth is not usually thought of as a sign of pre-eclampsia but it can indicate a failing placenta, which appears to be the source of the disease, and can be the first sign of the condition, particularly of early onset pre-eclampsia although less so of the disease occurring at term (Redman 1995). Slow growth is likely to be suspected on palpation and can be confirmed on ultrasound scan. Serial measurements of head circumference, abdominal circumference, femur and biparietal diameters are taken and plotted on fetal growth charts. However, these measurements are not helpful unless the pregnancy has been accurately dated in early pregnancy.

☐ Laboratory investigations

Blood test results can be valuable in making a diagnosis; they should include the following:

- Uric acid levels, which increase in pre-eclampsia, indicating impaired renal function (Redman *et al* 1976);

- Raised liver enzymes such as AST (plasma transaminase) can detect HELLP syndrome (see below) in pre-eclampsia (Weinstein 1982);

- Platelet counts fall in pre-eclampsia, demonstrating the platelet consumption seen in pre-eclampsia (Boneu *et al* 1980).

■ Symptoms

☐ Abdominal pain, vomiting and jaundice

Symptoms, such as epigastric pain, headaches and visual disturbances, the latter being highly noticeable for women, occur only at a late stage of the disease. The significance of abdominal pain and vomiting is often missed, particularly by family doctors who encounter such symptoms every day in their patients. The pain may easily be confused with heartburn, which is, of course, a very common problem of pregnancy. For this reason, it is important that all such complaints are not cursorily brushed aside. The epigastric pain of the HELLP syndrome is not burning in quality, does not spread upwards towards the throat, is associated with hepatic tenderness, may radiate through to the back and is not relieved by antacid (Weinstein 1982). Jaundice is a rare presentation of pre-eclampsia that is frequently misinterpreted and can be a sign of fulminating pre-eclampsia necessitating immediate delivery.

■ Complications of pre-eclampsia

☐ HELLP syndrome

The HELLP syndrome is one of the most important crises that can complicate pre-eclampsia. HELLP is an acronym for haemolysis, elevated liver enzymes and low platelets. These complications, the symptoms of which were described in the previous section, may occur with or without (ELLP syndrome) haemolysis. It usually presents with acute epigastric or right upper quadrant pain, and hepatic tenderness.

The syndrome may develop before or after delivery. In the 304 cases that were studied by Sibai (1990), 69 per cent occurred before delivery and 31 per cent afterwards. Amongst the antepartum group, 4 per cent developed the syndrome as early as 17–20 weeks gestation, and in 11 per cent it occurred at 21–26 weeks. There was 1 maternal death, 1 ruptured subcapsular haematoma of the liver, 5 cases of acute renal failure and 12 cases of disseminated intravascular coagulation (DIC). The findings underscore the importance of suspecting the presence of this syndrome in all pregnant women who complain of right upper quadrant abdominal pain, malaise, nausea or vomiting, even early in the second half of pregnancy.

Sibai (1990) found that several of the pregnancies were complicated with abruptio placentae, fetal distress, fetal growth retardation and fetal death during conservative management of the condition.

In the postpartum group, the time of onset of the manifestations ranged from a few hours to 6 days, the majority developing within 48 hours postpartum. Seventy-five patients (79 per cent) had evidence of pre-eclampsia before delivery; however, 21 per cent had no such evidence either before or during delivery (unheralded disease).

The typical presenting complaint of the HELLP syndrome is epigastric pain associated with malaise. The epigastric pain is often very severe, described by sufferers as the worst pain that they have ever experienced. Affected women are not uncommonly referred to general surgeons as suffering from an acute abdominal condition, for example acute cholecystitis (Weinstein 1982). Women who present with unexplained epigastric pain should be admitted to hospital as a matter of urgency even if there are no other signs of pre-eclampsia.

■ Eclampsia – the onset of convulsions

Eclampsia can occur before, during or after delivery and is a major cause of maternal or fetal mortality (DoH 1994). Eclamptic fits are triggered by abnormal activity in the nerve cells of the brain; when these cells are damaged, as they can be by the pre-eclamptic process, their highly organised activity can become so disturbed that it explodes into intense electrical discharges, which stimulate the convulsive movements. Eclamptic fits usually occur as the final complication of severe pre-eclampsia, but sometimes occur unexpectedly, without any evidence of preceding disturbances, although other signs of pre-eclampsia tend to appear at the same time as the fits (Redman & Walker 1992).

As previously mentioned, the BEST Study (Douglas & Redman 1994) established certain risk factors. Teenagers were three times more likely to suffer eclampsia than were older women, and women with multiple pregnancies were also significantly more susceptible. No increase was detected in women over the age of 34 years. Twenty-six of the 96 women with previous viable pregnancies had a history of pre-eclampsia, and one had a history of eclampsia. Thus 18 per cent of all cases were parous women with no previous history of pre-eclampsia or eclampsia.

The reduction in incidence in the UK between the 1920s and the 1970s occurred as antenatal care became universally available. This is shown by the fact that countries without effective antenatal screening programmes still have much higher incidence rates (Porapakkham 1979). Most cases in the study, however, occurred despite a normal frequency of antenatal assessments (70 per cent), and even after admission to hospital (77 per cent), which is not surprising since most of the cases occurred in relation to delivery and the puerperium. Furthermore, eclampsia was often (38 per cent) unheralded by hypertension and proteinuria.

For midwives in the community, the most important skill is of early detection of any of the signs of pre-eclampsia and early referral to the consultant unit. Paramedic teams in the ambulance service are now being trained to deal with an eclamptic fit in the home, and emergency services should be called if this occurs.

■ Recommendations for clinical practice in the light of currently available evidence

1. There is a need for midwives to assess the frequency of antenatal visits. In view of the research shown in this chapter, there is already a delay in visits between 20 and 28 weeks of gestation, and current suggestions that the duration could be longer should make midwives question the advisability of this.

2. A careful booking history should be taken at the onset of pregnancy, being aware of any increased risks for developing pre-eclampsia.

3. All routine antenatal checks must adhere to basic practice, ensuring that the blood pressure is measured and compared with the baseline

figure. The urine should be tested and checked for proteinuria. The pregnant woman should be weighed, on the same scales if possible, and the weight gain checked against previous visits. Recommendations that routine weighing can be abandoned need to be critically questioned.

4. Observe for signs of oedema and check carefully for any symptoms such as headache, visual disturbances or epigastric pain.

5. Early referral to hospital is essential if there is any reason for concern about the woman's condition.

6. Women with proteinuria and hypertension together must be admitted to hospital on the same day that the problem is detected. Women with unexplained epigastric pain should be assumed to have the HELLP syndrome until proved otherwise, and should also be admitted urgently.

7. Blood tests can confirm diagnosis. In high-risk women, there is a need for routine haematology and biochemistry to be taken at the booking visit to provide baseline measurements.

8. Women should know about pre-eclampsia. It can be a topic avoided at parentcraft classes for fear of alarming pregnant mothers, but it can be more frightening to develop a disease about which they know nothing.

■ Practice check

● How complete and considered is your routine antenatal check in the light of the previously mentioned research findings?

● Community midwives may know the women in their care well and be the first to hear of symptoms or detect facial oedema. What facilities do you have for fast communication between professionals, for advice or referral?

● How well do you listen to the women in your care? What response do they get from you if they describe unusual symptoms or if they feel unwell?

● What is your response to symptoms such as vomiting or 'heartburn'?

☐ Acknowledgements

Thank you to Miss Geraldine Gaffney for advising me on the construction of this chapter, to Miss Susan Sellers for rearranging the construction and to Professor Redman for his invaluable assistance with much of its content.

■ References

Abitbol MM 1969 Weight gain in pregnancy. American Journal of Obstetrics and Gynecology 104: 140–56

Baird D 1977 Epidemiological aspects of hypertensive pregnancy. Clinical Obstetrics and Gynaecology 4: 531–48

Boneu B, Fournie A, Sie P, Grandjean H, Bierme R, Pontonnier G 1980 Platelet production time, uricemia and some hemostasis tests in pre-eclampsia. European Journal of Obstetrics, Gynaecology and Reproductive Biology 11: 85–94

Boyd PA, Lindenbaum RH, Redman CWG 1987 Preeclampsia and trisomy 13: a possible association. Lancet ii: 425–7

Brosens I, Renaer M 1972 On the pathogenesis of placental infarcts in pre-eclampsia. Journal of Obstetrics and Gynaecology 79: 794–9

Brosens IA, Robertson WB, Dixon HG 1972 The role of the spiral arteries in the pathogenesis of pre-eclampsia. Obstetrics and Gynecology Annual 1: 177–91

Butler NR, Bonham DG 1963 Perinatal mortality. E and S Livingstone, Edinburgh, p87–100

Campbell DM, MacGillivray I 1985 Pre-eclampsia in second pregnancy. British Journal of Obstetrics and Gynaecology 82: 131–40

Chelsey LC, Annitto JE, Cosgrove RA 1968 The familial factor in toxaemia of pregnancy. Obstetrics and Gynecology 32: 303–11

Chun D, Braga C, Chow C, Lok L 1964 Clinical observations on some aspects of hydatidiform moles. Journal of Obstetrics and Gynaecology 71: 180–4

Cooper DW, Liston WA 1979 Genetic control of severe pre-eclampsia. Journal of Medical Genetics 16(6): 409–16

Department of Health, Welsh Office, Scottish Office Home and Health Department, Department of Health and Social Security, Northern Ireland 1994 Report on confidential enquiries into maternal deaths in the United Kingdom 1988–90. HMSO, London

DeWolf F, DeWolf Peeters C, Brosens I, Robertson WB 1980 The human placental bed: electron microscopic study of trophoblastic invasion of spiral arteries. American Journal of Obstetrics and Gynecology 137: 58–70

Douglas KA, Redman CWG 1994 Eclampsia in the United Kingdom. British Medical Journal 309: 1395–9

Gallery ED, Hunyor SN, Gyory AZ 1979 Plasma volume contraction: a significant factor in both pregnancy-associated hypertension (pre-eclampsia) and chronic hypertension in pregnancy. Quarterly Journal of Medicine 48: 593–602

Gallery ED, Delprado W, Gyory AZ 1981 Antihypertensive effect of plasma volume expansion in pregnancy-associated hypertension. Australian and New Zealand Journal of Medicine 11: 20–4

Gerretsen G, Huisjes HJ, Elema JD 1981 Morphological changes of the spiral arteries in the placental bed in relation to pre-eclampsia and fetal growth retardation. British Journal of Obstetrics and Gynaecology 88: 876–81

Groenendijk R, Trimbos JBMJ, Wallenberg HCS 1984 Hemodynamic measurements in preeclampsia: preliminary observations. American Journal of Obstetrics and Gynecology 150: 232–6

Highby K, Suiter CR, Phelps J, Siler-Khodr T, Langer O 1994 Normal values of urinary albumin and total protein excretion during pregnancy. American Journal of Obstetrics and Gynecology 171: 984–9

Jeffcoate NA, Scott JS 1959 Some observations on the placental factor in pregnancy toxaemia. American Journal of Obstetrics and Gynecology 77: 475–89

Khong TY, DeWolf F, Robertson WB, Brosens I 1986 Inadequate maternal vascular response to placentation in pregnancies complicated by pre-eclampsia and by small-for-gestational age infants. British Journal of Obstetrics and Gynaecology 93: 1049–59

MacGillivray I 1959 Some observations on the incidence of pre-eclampsia. Journal of Obstetrics and Gynaecology 65: 536–9

Naeye RL, Friedman EA 1979 Causes of perinatal death associated with gestational hypertension and proteinuria. American Journal of Obstetrics and Gynecology 133: 8–10

Page EW 1938 The relation between hydatid moles, relative ischemia of the gravid uterus, and the placental origin of eclampsia. American Journal of Obstetrics and Gynecology 37: 291–3

Pijnenborg R, Robertson WB, Brosens I, Dixon G 1981 Review article: trophoblast invasion and the establishment of haemochorial placentation in man and laboratory animals. Placenta 2: 71–91

Porapakkham S 1979 An epidemiologic study of eclampsia. Obstetrics and Gynecology 54(1): 26–30

Redman CWG 1989 Hypertension in pregnancy. In Turnbull SA, Chamberlain G (eds) Obstetrics. Churchill Livingstone, Edinburgh, p515–41

Redman CWG 1993 The placenta, pre-eclampsia and chronic villitis. In Redman CWG, Sargent IL, Starkey PM (eds) The human placenta. Blackwell Scientific, Oxford, p433–67

Redman CWG 1995 Medical disorders of pregnancy. In De Swiet M (ed.) Medical disorders in obstetric practice, 3rd edn. Blackwell Scientific, Oxford, Ch 6

Redman CWG, Roberts JM 1993 Management of pre-eclampsia. Lancet 341: 1451

Redman CWG, Sargent IL 1993 The immunology of pre-eclampsia. In: Chaouat G (ed.) Immunology of pregnancy. CRC Press, London, p205–30

Redman CWGR, Walker I 1992 Pre-eclampsia: the facts. Oxford University Press, Oxford

Redman CWG, Beilin LJ, Bonnar J 1976 Renal function in pre-eclampsia. Journal of Clinical Pathology 10 (supplement): 91–4

Roberts JM, Redman CWG 1993 Pre-eclampsia: more than pregnancy-induced hypertension. Lancet 341: 1447–51

Roberts JM, Taylor RN, Musci TJ, Rogers GM, Hubel CA, McLaughlin MK 1989 Preeclampsia: an endothelial cell disorder. American Journal of Obstetrics and Gynecology 161: 1200–4

Robertson WB, Brosens I, Dixon G 1975 Uteroplacental vascular pathology. European Journal of Obstetrics, Gynaecology and Reproductive Biology 5: 47–65

Robillard PY, Hulsey TC, Perianin J, Janky E, Miri EH, Papiernik E 1994 Association of pregnancy-induced hypertension with duration of sexual cohabitation before conception. Lancet 344(8928): 973–5

Scott JS 1958 Pregnancy toxaemia associated with hydrops foetalis, hydatidiform mole and hydramnios. Journal of Obstetrics and Gynaecology 65: 689–701

Sheehan HL, Lynch JB 1973 Pathology of toxaemia of pregnancy. Churchill Livingstone, Edinburgh, p 328–474

Shennan AH, Hallighan A, Gupta M, Taylor D, DeSwiet M 1995 Indirect blood pressure measurement in pregnancy: reproducibility of Korotkoff phase IV and V. Abstract, International Society for the Study of Hypertension in Pregnancy, Leuven, Belgium, 21 July 1995

Sibai BM 1990 The HELLP syndrome (hemolysis, elevated liver enzymes, and low platelets): much ado about nothing? American Journal of Obstetrics and Gynecology 162: 311–16

Sibai BM, McCubbin JH, Anderson GD, Lipshitz J, Dilts PVJ 1991 Eclampsia. I. Observations from 67 recent cases. Obstetrics and Gynecology 77: 331–7

Taylor HC, Tillman AJ, Blanchard J 1954 Fetal losses in hypertension and pre-eclampsia. Obstetrics and Gynaecology 3: 225–39

Weinstein L 1982 Syndrome of hemolysis, elevated liver enzymes, low platelet count; a severe consequence of hypertension on pregnancy. American Journal of Obstetrics and Gynecology 142: 159–67

■ Suggested further reading

Douglas KA, Redman CWG 1994 Eclampsia in the United Kingdom. British Medical Journal 309: 1395–9

Redman CWG 1995 Medical disorders of pregnancy. In DeSwiet M (ed.) Medical disorders in obstetric practice, 3rd edn. Blackwell Scientific, Oxford, Ch 6

Redman CWG, Walker I 1992 Pre-eclampsia: the facts. Oxford Medical Publications, Oxford

Chapter 9

Marketing midwifery services

Kathleen King

When questioning a group of midwives about their definition of marketing, I received a mixed response. Common answers were 'Advertising and promotion' and 'Selling'. More cynical respondents believed it to be about 'Getting people to buy things they don't really want or need'. Little wonder then that, with the arrival of the internal market in the NHS, midwives have often taken a reluctant interest in the subject. However, the reorganisation of the NHS as a business, largely driven by economic principles, requires all services, including midwifery, to bid for scarce resources, justify expenditure and improve efficiency. Midwifery needs to convince potential buyers of the value and potential of its services and convince policy makers of its important role in the future of maternity services (Hauxwell & Rees 1995). Marketing theories have much to offer midwifery service providers, and many professional groups within the NHS have already accepted their importance.

This chapter takes a closer look at the special nature of the maternity services that confronts the service provider with particular problems. It offers a working definition of marketing as a philosophy and a management tool and illustrates how marketing can help providers of maternity services better to meet the needs of their purchasers and users. A conceptual model of service quality aims to encourage a critical review of the service quality levels within the reader's own organisation.

■ It is assumed that you are already aware of the following:

● The general principles of the purchaser–provider split in the NHS;

and the key content of

● *Working for patients* (DoH 1989);

- *The patient's charter* (DoH 1992);
- *Changing childbirth* (DoH 1993);
- *Maternity services charter* (DoH 1994);
- *Changing childbirth update* (DoH 1995).

■ Who is 'the customer'?

At the core of every marketing theory lies the concept of the customer, and a crucial task for service providers is to determine who their customers are. This, however, is not as straightforward as it may seem. Recent reforms in the NHS have separated providers from purchasers of services. This means that providers now have two types of customer: the purchasers or buyers, mainly GP fundholders and District Health Authorities (DHAs), and the users; they are therefore faced with a 'customer chain' (Stokes 1994). This may lead to complex and sometimes difficult decisions, since the requirements of purchasers may well be different from the needs and wishes of the users. For instance, the DHA may want to contain costs by reducing the length of stay in hospital of mother and child, whereas some mothers might like to stay longer to enjoy the relative peace on the ward and the reassuring presence of health care staff. Meeting the needs of the users, at the expense of the purchasers, could well encourage the purchasers to take their business elsewhere. Meanwhile, dissatisfied users can lead to customer complaints and again may adversely affect the competitiveness of the organisation. Service providers need to give careful consideration to the needs of both purchasers and users and attempt to strike a balance between the two. Involving both purchasers and users in the process of the service design and specification and in resolving discrepancies between purchaser and user needs, can avoid both controversies and making promises that cannot be delivered. This issue will be returned to when we consider the service quality model.

■ The nature of services

It is frequently argued that services have unique characteristics that differentiate them from goods and manufactured products (Payne 1993) and that these characteristics can have a profound impact on service delivery and marketing, especially from the users' perspective. Before discussing the potential of marketing for midwifery services, we need to consider the special features of services and the implications of these for the service provider (Sheaff 1991; King's Fund 1993; NHS Management Executive 1993).

Four key characteristics of services are intangibility, inseparability, heterogeneity and perishability (Mudie & Cottam 1993). Each of those features needs to be seen as existing on a continuum.

☐ Intangibility

Services cannot generally be seen, felt, tried or tested before being bought. The challenge is for the service organisation to provide the purchaser with tangible evidence wherever possible. Trusts can provide purchasers with detailed maternity service specifications and documentation outlining the services available to women, and can pay careful attention to the tangible aspect of their services, such as the ward environment, personnel and equipment. An important implication of intangibility is that users tend to rely more heavily on personal recommendation from their peer group than they would for the purchase of goods. In the UK, people tend to be poor at complaining to the service provider when they receive bad service (Payne 1993) but are likely to take their business elsewhere while spreading the bad news to an average of nine or ten others (Dobree & Page 1991).

☐ Inseparability

Goods are produced, stored and finally sold and consumed. Services are, on the contrary, first sold and then produced and used simultaneously. For the production of maternity services, the user has to be physically present. This has important implications for service quality, especially as perceived by users. The conduct of every member of staff, from the telephone operator to midwives and consultants, is part of the users' (women and their family and friends) experience and will inform their perception of the service quality. Therefore, careful selection and training, especially of contact personnel, are important for quality assurance.

Another implication of inseparability is the fact that users have an impact on each other's experience of the service. 'Impatient patients' in the waiting room, whiling away time complaining about the service, or screaming children may turn an otherwise problem free check-up into a nerveracking experience. Attention to detail, such as up to date literature, refreshment facilities and the provision of toys in waiting areas, can be a cost effective measure contributing greatly to the perceived service quality and adding a competitive edge over other providers.

☐ **Heterogeneity**

The simultaneous production and use of a service unavoidably leads to variability in performance. The quality of midwifery services will vary not only depending on which midwife provides them, but also for one particular midwife from day to day. Factors such as professional and interpersonal skills create variances between midwives. Stress, fatigue and interpersonal chemistry between midwife and woman can account for intrapersonal variations. This can make the standardisation of services and quality control particularly difficult. Setting clear service standards and specifications, determining causes of variability and seeking continuous feedback from users may help to reduce unwanted variations. However, too much emphasis on standards may lead to rigidity and fragmentation, distracting attention from what really matters: the total process experienced by the user (Christopher *et al* 1991).

☐ **Perishability**

Services cannot be stored for later use. Unoccupied beds in a maternity ward cannot be reclaimed, and having staff on duty on a half empty ward is a very expensive waste of resources. Careful activity analysis, taking seasonal variations into account, is a useful tool for producing well-balanced staff rotas. Many NHS Trusts are facing the reverse problem: occupation of wards is almost continuously at full capacity, with no room for expansion to meet the demand. Development of community services not only allows expansion of market share, but is also within the spirit of government guidelines in the *Patient's charter* (DoH 1992) and the *Maternity services charter* (DoH 1994).

Bateson (1992) summarises the implications of the above service characteristics by pointing out that, in service organisations, the *inanimate* environment (buildings and equipment), all contact personnel, the part of the organisation invisible to the user (support staff and systems) as well as other customers all have an impact on the service experience.

■ **What is marketing?**

The UK Institute of Marketing defines marketing as 'The management process responsible for identifying, anticipating and satisfying customer requirements profitably'. Marketing is both a philosophy and a function in an organisation (Stokes 1994).

☐ A philosophy of customer orientation

Adoption of this philosophy means that everything an organisation does, the service it delivers, the direction it takes, is driven by what its customers want, because they are the *'raison d'être'* of the organisation. Customers are consulted about their needs, and services are developed to meet those needs. Continuous monitoring of customer satisfaction ensures that the organisation remains flexible in its response to changing customer needs. This is a fundamentally different approach from the so-called *service orientation* often found with professionals; because of their high levels of expertise and specialised knowledge, professionals tend to have very firm views on what is best for the customer and to concentrate on providing the service or treatment *they* believe to be appropriate (Hunt & Symonds 1995). Such was the trend to bring women into hospital for their labour, which was inspired more by the concern of the medical and midwifery professions for safety and convenience than by the needs and wants of the mothers and their families. The government has endorsed the importance of a marketing philosophy in the *Maternity services charter*, emphasising pregnant women's rights and the choices they can expect to make under the *Patient's charter* (DoH 1992).

☐ A management function

An organisation's vision and mission, based on a marketing philosophy, can lead to a truly customer focused statement of purpose or mission. This mission needs to be translated into key objectives for the organisation, and strategies need to be specified that will help the organisation to meet those objectives (Stokes 1994). Developing a strategy that allows the organisation to compete with other providers requires a careful analysis of:

- The environment in which the organisation operates;

- Its competitors in the market;

- Its own resources, skills and competences.

This process, the so-called 'marketing audit' (McDonald 1995), is iterative and complex. The external environment (social, technological, economic and political developments) cannot easily be influenced, but nevertheless needs to be understood and incorporated in the organisation's strategy and tactics – the detailed plans for implementing the strategy. Excellent organisations continuously monitor changes in their environment and adapt their strategies to make the most of new opportunities (Kotler, 1988, 1991).

The ingredients that make up an organisation's programme for

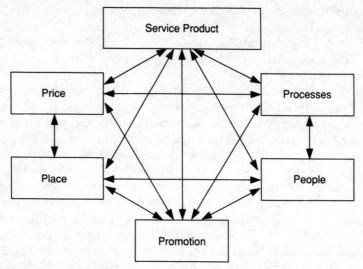

Figure 9.1   The marketing mix for services (adapted from Payne 1993)

delivering its strategy are called the marketing mix. Traditionally the
marketing mix covered four elements: product, price, place and promotion,
each of which comprises a collection of subactivities. For example, place
includes the location and channels through which the service will be
delivered (Payne 1993). If the elements of the marketing mix are not
comprehensive, a gap might occur between the market requirements and
the organisation's services on offer. Consequently, many authors have
argued that a different marketing mix is needed for services. Payne's
(1993) model added several new elements to the marketing mix; here we
will use a simplification of the final model, using only the extra factors of
people and processes (Fig. 9.1). This provides a useful framework for
building an integrated marketing strategy. The service provider needs to
consider the individual elements and ensure that they are mutually congruent in order to develop a consistent marketing strategy. We shall discuss each element in turn and apply it to midwifery service provisions.

The service product

What are your customers getting? The answer to this question is not as
straightforward as it may seem. For example, is a person buying a Cartier
watch purchasing a time measuring device or a status symbol? There is
an important distinction to be made between the service characteristics
and the benefits as they are perceived by the customer. Is, for example, a
DHA buying your services looking for value for money, for an excellent
reputation or for the most conveniently located provider? Which particular benefits make your service more attractive to both purchasers and
users than that of your competitors? A thorough understanding of your

service from the perspective of your purchasers is essential for the development of your services, as well as for your strategy regarding other aspects of your marketing mix.

Place

Location is concerned with where an organisation's operations and staff are to be found (Payne 1993). As with all other aspects of the marketing mix, it is important to consider this element from the customers' perspective. In maternity services, there are generally two types of interaction:

- The women come to the service provider;
- The service provider goes to the women.

When women come to the hospital, location becomes a very important aspect of the service. A key consideration is the impact of the environment on the users (Bateson 1992). The configuration of the hospital, the decor, its location in the catchment area, easy access by public or private transport, parking facilities, and so on are all part of the service and need careful attention. Another important question is whether there is sufficient space to meet the needs of the catchment area; is there room for expansion?

When the maternity service provider goes to the women, location is equally important. Clinics need to be established within easy reach of the women's homes and providers need to be easily contactable, to be able to reach the women at short notice, to keep in regular contact and to provide back-up in case of an emergency. A key question regarding *place* for the maternity service is the preference of the user, in this case the woman and her family.

Price

In a business environment, the pricing strategy is a key element in positioning the service in the market: high prices may be charged for an exclusive, high-quality niche in the market; moderate prices allow the provider to reach a larger number of customers with a more modest service. Owing to restrictions on pricing strategies in the NHS (prices have to be cost based) and to limited funds available to purchasers, providers price their services as competitively as possible in order to maintain their share of the market. This places an increasing onus on cost structures and value for money, limiting the options for exclusive services that would require prohibitive prices. Again, careful analysis of purchaser requirements and their price sensitivity is essential.

Promotion

The role of a promotion strategy is to inform, persuade or remind customers about the services being offered (Bateson 1992). The service provider needs to define the target audience, determine promotion objectives, develop the message and select the appropriate communication channels. Different communication strategies will need to be developed for different audiences, depending on their varying needs. For example, promotion of a maternity unit to GP fundholders will employ different information and phraseology concerning the potential users, and promotion to GPs outside the catchment area might well emphasise different service aspects from promotional material for local GPs.

In high-contact services such as midwifery, communications need to be directed at employees as well as at customers. When customers buy 'the performance of employees', promotion needs to be concerned not only with encouraging customers to buy, but also with encouraging employees to perform (George & Berry 1981).

Personal selling is an important channel for maternity services promotion. Providers need to establish and maintain good working relationships with current and prospective purchasers and keep them informed of and involved in new developments (Payne & Ballantyne 1991). Research shows that personal recommendation is one of the most important information sources for services promotion (Payne 1993): users attach importance to the word of mouth endorsement by their peer group because of the intangible and variable nature of services. Maternity service providers can capitalise on this tool by using testimonials in their promotion material and incorporating feedback in a comprehensive complaints procedure: 'If you're happy tell others, if you're not tell us' (Mudie & Cottam, 1994: 175). Complaints need to be dealt with quickly and effectively.

People

People are the key asset in a services organisation: any service is only as good as the people delivering it. Because of the users' involvement in service delivery, every employee can have an impact on the perceived service quality: the perception of a maternity unit employing excellent midwives and consultants will be adversely influenced by unfriendly or disorganised support personnel, such as receptionists, porters or cleaners. Providing an excellent service to users requires every individual and every department in the organisation to provide and receive excellent service to and from each other. As highlighted in 'Promotion' above, all employees need to work together in a way that is congruent with the organisation's objectives, strategies and goals, especially in high-contact services such as midwifery, in order to give a consistent message to the outside world (Payne 1993).

Employees can be seen as internal customers (Bateson 1992). For example, midwives are supported by administrative and maintenance staff in their delivery of a high-quality service. Attracting, motivating, training and retaining high-quality employees is a key task for any service organisation. Service organisations need to develop jobs and reward systems that will satisfy individual needs, as the best people are attracted to work for organisations that are seen to be good employers.

Processes

Processes involve the procedures, tasks, schedules and all activities and routines by which a service is delivered. People are crucial in the effective delivery of services, but no amount of employee effort will be able to overcome ineffective process performance (Payne 1993). For example, a mother, although grateful for the excellent support of the midwives and medical team during a complicated pregnancy, may become increasingly dissatisfied at having to wait long periods of time to be seen in the ante-natal clinic. Making an inventory of all processes involved in the service delivery and breaking down the processes into logical steps and sequences facilitates its analysis and control (Shostack 1987). Well-planned and structured processes can add to improved cost effectiveness as well as to service quality. They may give the provider a competitive edge over less efficient competitors.

Effective marketing management requires not only attention to every element of the marketing mix, but also careful consideration of the integration of the mix. Every factor needs to support and enhance the others: promotion needs to emphasise the key merits of people, processes and place; processes and people need to be appropriate for the location element; and so on. For example, an NHS Trust developing a community maternity service as a result of insufficient capacity on its maternity ward and the increasing request for home births, will need to develop a dedicated marketing mix for its community services by defining its key promotional targets and message, recruiting the right people to deliver the service, developing processes for its smooth delivery and, in co-operation with its purchasers, developing an effective pricing strategy. This entire process should be underpinned by a marketing philosophy: the most efficient, quality service will only be effective and achieve organisational success if it meets the needs of its customers (Owens & McGill 1993).

■ Service quality

In the analysis of service characteristics and the marketing mix, we have already identified some potential difficulties in developing and maintaining service quality. Service quality is also a very elusive concept. Purchasers and users often find it difficult to articulate their precise requirements, and providers, especially professionals, tend to focus on what they believe is best for the client. Quality, however, is in the eyes of the beholder. The quality of the service, as *perceived* by the client (compared with the expectations of the client), rather than quality as perceived by the provider, will eventually dictate whether or not an organisation will receive repeat business and remain competitive (Gronroos 1980).

Parasuraman *et al* (1985) developed a model of service quality that helps the service provider to identify potential gaps between what customers expect and the service they perceive they get. This model identifies five potential gaps. Gaps 1–4 are all shortfalls within the organisation; these contribute to gap 5, which is the quality shortfall as perceived by the customer. We will take a closer look at this model, giving examples from the perspective of women using maternity services. The model is, however, equally applicable to service quality as perceived by purchasers.

☐ **Gap 1: Discrepancy between consumer expectation and management perception of consumer expectation**

Parasuraman *et al* (1985) propose that the size of this gap is a function of:

- The amount of market research undertaken and the extent to which it focuses on service quality issues;

- The quality and extent of upward communications in the organisation;

- The number of layers between customer contact personnel and top managers.

In other words, the less feedback that management receives from users, either directly or indirectly, the more likely this gap is to widen.

- *An NHS Trust had invested in smart new uniforms for the midwives. From communications between midwives and women, management discovered that most women considered the uniforms of midwives to be irrelevant or unimportant and would have much rather seen the money invested in upgrading some of the facilities on the maternity ward.*

- *A midwife encouraged a woman to keep her children at home for the expected date of the delivery. It only emerged later that the woman would have preferred her children to stay with her mother but had felt too embarrassed to express this.*

☐ **Gap 2: Discrepancy between management perception and service quality specification**

A number of factors may contribute to this gap: resource limitations, management's commitment to service quality, task standardisation, the existence of a formal process to set service quality objectives and the extent to which managers believe that customer expectations can be met.

- *Mothers expressed the need for privacy after the delivery, but the NHS Trust Board perceived the provision of single rooms to be too expensive.*

- *Women may interpret continuity of care as being cared for by the named midwife at least 90 per cent of the time, whereas management may consider 50 per cent of the time to be satisfactory.*

☐ **Gap 3: Discrepancy between service quality specification and service delivery**

This gap may be called the service performance gap and is the extent to which service specifications are not met by the staff delivering the service. Effective interdisciplinary teamwork, co-operation between management and employees, the extent to which employees feel valued and committed to their work, the ability of employees to perform their tasks, the perceived clarity of goals and expectations, and the absence of conflict between expectations of customers and expectations of the organisation can all contribute to closing this gap.

- *In times of temporary staff shortage, an NHS Trust may have to employ bank staff, who may need time to settle into the team and adjust to the routine on the ward.*

- *A maternity unit may have waiting times specified as a maximum of 30 minutes, while in reality women regularly have to wait for over an hour before being seen by the midwife or consultant.*

☐ **Gap 4: Discrepancy between service delivery and external communications**

Exaggerated promises in external communications and/or the absence of clear information about the services provided can affect the customers' perception of service quality. This gap depends on both external and internal communications. Contact personnel need to be aware of service specifications and of communication with customers. Because they deliver the actual service, they need to be involved in the promotion strategy of the organisation. If there is a tendency to overpromise when agreeing service specifications with purchasers in order to win the contract, consultants and midwives will find that they cannot deliver the specified service, despite their best efforts.

- *In the Maternity Services Charter (DoH 1994) mothers are promised that babies can be looked after in a nursery. In reality, women are strongly encouraged to look after their baby because of security risks and to aid 'bonding' and breastfeeding.*

● *The promotional material of a community service promised women that they would be cared for by no more than two different midwives. However, holiday and sick leave of midwives meant that women could be visited by any midwife out of a team of five.*

☐ **Gap 5: Discrepancy between the expected service and the perceived service**

The service that customers expect to receive depends on their personal needs and past experience, promotion by the organisation and word of mouth promotion by other service users. If, because of any combination of the above factors, expectations are too high, the customer is likely to be disappointed. This gap again emphasises the need for clear communication and accurate information passed from the service provider to the customer.

● *Because of the enthusiastic recommendation of fertility treatment by a consultant, a woman and her husband were left sorely disappointed when they eventually had to give up after a number of unsuccessful treatments.*

● *Promotional material had left a woman totally unprepared for the run down, dilapidated condition of the maternity areas in her local hospital.*

Delivering consistently excellent service quality is a difficult, and sometimes moving, target. Obtaining regular feedback from customers, positively encouraging and rewarding it (small prize draws have been known to make all the difference to return rates for questionnaires), clear internal and external communications and good employee relations, can all contribute to improved quality and competitiveness.

■ **Practice check**

● Do you have any mechanisms in place to monitor the needs of your purchasers and users? If you do, how does the obtained information inform current and future practice? If you do not, how might you establish a means of obtaining this information?

● Is there a mission statement for the area in which you work? Do you find yourself in harmony with it?

● Do you have a personal mission statement/philosophy of care?

- How do you keep informed about developments of other maternity service providers who are potential competitors?

- Applying Parasuraman *et al*'s (1985) model, what do you consider some major strengths and weaknesses of your organisation regarding service quality? What could you recommend for improving the service quality?

- Apply the marketing mix to one of your services (for instance antenatal care or delivery). Do you find consistency between the various elements of the marketing mix?

- Design an effective promotional strategy for the purchasers and users of one of your services.

■ References

Bateson J 1992 Managing services marketing: text and readings. Dryden, Chicago

Department of Health 1989 Working for patients. HMSO, London

Department of Health 1992 The patient's charter. HMSO, London

Department of Health 1993 Changing childbirth update 1. HMSO, London

Department of Health 1994 Maternity services charter. HMSO, London

Dobree J, Page AS 1991 Unleashing the power of service brands in the 1990s. Management Decisions 28: 6

George WR and Berry LL 1981 Guidelines for the advertising of services. Business Horizons 24 (4): 52–6. In Payne A 1993 The essence of services marketing. Prentice Hall, Hemel Hempstead p381–5

Gronroos C 1980 Designing a long range marketing strategy for services. Long Range Planning 13: 36–42. In Bateson J 1992 Managing services marketing: text and readings. Dryden, Chicago, p458–67

Hauxwell B, Rees C 1995 Marketing midwifery's future. British Journal of Midwifery 3: 6

Hunt S, Symonds A 1995 The social meaning of midwifery. Macmillan, Basingstoke

King's Fund Centre 1993 Maternity care: choice, continuity and change: consensus statement. King's Fund Centre, London

Kotler P 1988 Marketing management. Prentice Hall, Englewood Cliffs, NJ

Kotler P 1991 Marketing management: analysis, planning, implementation and control. Prentice Hall, Englewood Cliffs, NJ

McDonald M 1995 Marketing plans: how to prepare them, how to use them. Butterworth–Heinemann, Oxford

Mudie P, Cottam A 1993 The management and marketing of services. Butterworth–Heinemann, Oxford

NHS Management Executive 1993 Market testing in the NHS: revised guidance. HMSO, London

Owens J, McGill J 1993 Marketing in the NHS: putting the patients first. NAHAT, Birmingham

Parasuraman A, Zeithalm V A, Berry LL 1985 A conceptual model of service quality and its implications for future research. Journal of Marketing 49: 41–50. In Bateson J 1992 Managing services marketing: text and readings. Dryden, Chicago, p507–20

Payne A 1993 The essence of services marketing. Prentice Hall, Hemel Hempstead

Payne A, Ballantyne D 1991 Relationship marketing: bringing customer service, quality and marketing together. Butterworth–Heinemann, Oxford

Sheaff R 1991 Marketing for health services: a framework for communications evaluation and total quality management. Open University Press, Milton Keynes

Shostack GL 1987 Service positioning through structural change. Journal of Marketing 51: 34–43. In Payne A 1993 The essence of services marketing. Prentice Hall, Hemel Hempstead, p169–71

Stokes D 1994 Discovering marketing: an active learning approach. DP Publications, London

■ Suggested further reading

Baxter-Derrington P 1995 Getting your message across. (Principles and process of marketing.) Nursing Standard 9: 20–3

Dickinson E 1995 Using marketing principles for healthcare development. Quality in Health Care 4(1): 40–4

Hobbs L 1993 Independent midwifery. Books for Midwives Press, Manchester

Hunt SC 1995 Marketing: a new concept for midwifery education. British Journal of Healthcare Management 1(9): 441–4

McLeish B 1995 Successful marketing strategies for nonprofit organizations. John Wiley, Chichester

Whitcroft M 1995 Marketing: hard sell. (Relevance of marketing to NHS purchasers and providers.) Health Service Journal 105: 30–1

Index